OMAD FASTING

How Intermittent Fasting With One Meal a Day Can Maximize
Your Weight Loss

(The Ultimate Guide on How You Can Activate Autophagy)

Marcus Ross

Published by Alex Howard

Omad Fasting: How Intermittent Fasting With One Meal a Day Can Maximize Your Weight Loss (The Ultimate Guide on How You Can Activate Autophagy)

ISBN 978-1-77485-008-4

Legal & Disclaimer

The information contained in this book is not designed to replace or take the place of any form of medicine or professional medical advice. The information in this book has been provided for educational and entertainment purposes only.

Table of contents

Part 1

Introduction: How Would It Feel to Be Free?

How many diets have you been on in your life? Have you lost count? Do you beat yourself up when you fall off an eating plan? How many times have you told yourself *"this time* it will be different"? Believe me, I completely understand. I've battled with my weight since I was a child. Up until a few years ago, I felt trapped in a cycle of starting a new diet; telling myself that I'd stick with it this time; falling off the plan; being mad at myself; eating more; gaining the weight back; being convinced I had to do something about my weight; finding out about a new diet ...and then I'd start the cycle over again. Can you relate to this?

You might feel like I did at that time. I felt desperate to change – but after countless attempts (with only short-lived positive results), my cycle of failure left me feeling hopeless that things could ever change permanently.

What if you could trade in that hopeless feeling for an expectation that you can and will succeed? And not just short-term success, but a lasting total body and health transformation?

How would it feel to be free? Free from doubts; free from failure; free from disappointment and free from

2

the all-too-familiar diet restrictions? Sounds pretty incredible, right?

At this point, you might be a bit skeptical. *Every* diet book on the market tells us *"This* is the answer you've been looking for!" So, I can understand your hesitation. I felt exactly the same way before I discovered intermittent fasting. How could this be different than any other approach to weight loss?

I was burnt out on dieting. I didn't want to try again. I thought if every diet eventually ended in disaster, why should I bother trying anymore?

Around that time, a friend of mine discovered intermittent fasting and was raving about it. Although it sounded interesting, initially I wouldn't even consider it as an option because I wasn't interested in going on another diet.

When I saw the results that my friend was getting, I was amazed. The extra pounds seemed to melt off of her and she radiated with confidence. Even though my walls were up, I started to do more research on the topic. I read a few books on intermittent fasting and was blown away. Could it be true that there was a way that I could successfully and sustainably reach my fat-loss goals? I had my doubts. But it sounded so different from everything else I've tried over the years. I realized I had another try in me.

I started practicing intermittent fasting and was fascinated at how the pounds seemed to effortlessly come off. Where had this way of eating been all my life?

It ends up that it's been around much longer than me (I am 50 years old) but it had fallen out of popularity in recent years. This is mainly due to the fact that modern society (in general) has lost sight of the immense benefits of "less". We've turned into a people always desiring "more".

In recent years, the idea of "less" has been increasing in popularity again. With concepts such as minimalism, decluttering and downsizing becoming more mainstream, we are starting to embrace the same ideas around our eating behaviors. Do we consume meals and snacks all day long because we should? Or because it's what our culture finds acceptable? Is it simply a habit? It's time to question what we think we know. Especially if the ideas we've been hanging onto haven't been serving us. I didn't even question my old view of requiring several meals a day. I thought it was a fact - it turns out that it is not.

I have tried (and enjoyed) many different types of intermittent fasting. I'll cover some of the different ways to practice it in Chapter 1. But my favorite has always been the One Meal A Day approach. Instead of restricting the amount of food (number of calories) or types of foods (i.e. no carbs or no fat), it simply restricts the time that you eat the foods you choose. There are no other limitations! This is a liberating discovery. You can eat the foods you desire (with no restriction on the amount) at a certain time of day. That's it! There are no other diet rules to remember. You can finally be truly free.

This book is designed as a quick-start guide that will get you going on your One Meal A Day plan as soon as possible. It's packed with all the basics to launch your successful journey.

I'm thrilled for the opportunity to pass along the information that has helped me to escape the diet/weight-gain cycle. I hope you're excited as well.

If you're still hesitant, that's ok. Just keep reading. I hope and pray that you will discover what I did – there actually is a different way! One that is simple and one that *works* for the long-haul. Now let's jump in to the fun!

Chapter 1: What Is OMAD?

Let's start with the basics. Fasting simply means: willingly abstaining from food (or calorie-containing beverages) for a specified amount of time. There are many different ways that people practice intermittent fasting (sometimes referred to as "IF"). There is no one "right" way to go about it. Some popular examples of different ways to practice fasting are:

16:8 Fasting

The person will refrain from eating or drinking calorie-containing beverages for 16 hours every day. They consume all their food in an 8-hour period.

20:4 Fasting (Sometimes Called The Warrior Diet)

The person following this plan will refrain from eating for 20 hours every day. They consume all their food in a 4-hour period.

5:2 Fasting

Just when you thought you had the number pattern figured out, I'm throwing 5:2 into the mix! 5:2 fasting indicates that the person will eat "normally" for 5 days out of the week and will abstain from food for 2 days a week. Typically, the fasting days are not consecutive. An example of this would be going without food every

Tuesday and Thursday – but eating regularly the other 5 days out of the week.

Alternate Day Fasting

A person following an alternative-day fasting regimen would eat "normally" on one day and fast for the next day. Additionally, some people add in one 500-calorie meal on their fast days while following this plan.

There are countless ways to observe intermittent fasting. These are just a few examples. The main aspect that they all have in common is that it is a pattern or rhythm of eating. To establish this rhythm, the person who is fasting will typically eat their food during the same time-period every day. This is also known as an "eating window".

An example of this would be someone following a 20:4 fasting schedule eating their food between the hours of 4 and 8 p.m. every day. Therefore, that person's daily "eating window" would be 4 p.m. – 8 p.m.

Please note: there is definitely room for flexibility and special occasions when you are following an intermittent fasting routine. But it is most beneficial to stay within a relatively consistent eating window to gain the most benefit from your fasts.

Here it is. The one you've been waiting for! The One Meal A Day Diet is also known by its acronym O.M.A.D. (or simply OMAD).

In my opinion, the One Meal A Day Diet is superior to all other ways of practicing fasting because you'll be enjoying the benefits of a maximum daily fasting time (allowing you to lose more weight or lose at a faster rate) while also allowing you to eat every day.

Plus, when you eat, you'll be able to eat whatever you want with (almost) no restrictions on the amount of food you can have! I say "almost" because everyone is different. One person may be able to eat unlimited portions and dessert every day, and another might need to limit that to a couple of times a week. We'll discuss this more in Chapter 4.

The bottom line is that you will no longer have to count calories ...or carbs ...or fat grams, etc. For the most part, you can eat what you want, in the amounts that you desire. How freeing would that be? You won't have to worry about what you "can" or "can't" have. You can simply enjoy yourself and your food. When friends or family invite you out, you won't have to choose between them and going off your diet. You can finally eat like a non-dieting person, while seeing amazing weight-loss results! Does this sound too good to be true? It's not.

People are rediscovering the incredible benefits of the ancient art of fasting. This is no fad. There is a reason why it's gaining momentum and popularity – because it WORKS.

OMAD is also sometimes referred to as 23:1 – meaning, you consume all of your food for the day within one hour. If only eating in a one-hour time period sounds impossible, I assure you it's not. You're most likely drawing off of experiences you've had in the past. Who hasn't skipped a meal, only to be ravenous later in the day? Because you've lived it before, you can't imagine feeling that same restriction (and subsequent "I-want-to-eat-everything-in-sight" feeling) day after day. Hang in there. Don't give up now. I promise you that it will not feel like that every day.

There are many factors that add up to the negative feelings and reactions we've had in the past after skipping one or more meals. Some of them are biological and some are habitual. We'll get deeper into that in the next chapter. For now, please just trust me when I say that once you get used to your new routine, you won't believe how easy it is to skip the other meals you used to eat.

It's best to keep this hour at approximately the same time every day. So, if it's important to you to eat dinner with your family, have your OMAD meal between 5 p.m. – 6 p.m. If your job requires you to take lunch or breakfast meetings, it would make more sense to choose an earlier time of day.

Although there has been much discussion and debate within the diet and weight loss community over what the best time of day to eat is – my opinion is there is no "correct" time. The time of day that is best to eat is the one that YOU can consistently stick with. In the past, I've eaten my one meal at dinner. More recently, I've switched it to mid-day. I find that only having to wait till lunch is easier for me during the day. When I have a filling meal that sustains me (which is the goal), by the time I'm starting to feel a bit hungry again, it's time to go to bed.

I want to stress that this is personal preference. Once you get used to eating one daily meal, you can try different times of the day and see what works best for you. I don't suggest playing with the times too early into your journey. Consistency in the beginning will help you more easily adjust to your new plan.

In the next chapter, we'll uncover the benefits of intermittent fasting. Not only can it help you lose weight easily and safely, but it can also transform your health and your outlook on life. Let's get to the good stuff...

Chapter 2: The Amazing Benefits of Intermittent Fasting

Intermittent fasting not only can turn your body into a fat-burning machine, but it also has countless health benefits. Plus, it can save you money and actually give you more time in your day to do the things you need to accomplish (or have always wanted to do)!

Fasting Benefits

According to intermittent fasting expert, Dr. Jason Fung, just a few of the health benefits derived from fasting are as follows:

- Weight/fat loss

- Lowering of blood insulin and blood sugar levels

- Increased energy

- Improved blood cholesterol levels

- Improved mental clarity

- Increased cellular cleansing, due to autophagy

- Increased growth hormone

- Reduced inflammation

- Possible reversal of type 2 diabetes

Although most of the benefits included in the list above are self-explanatory, there are a few that might not seem that exciting at first glance. Let's take a deeper look at a couple of them.

Autophagy

The word autophagy was derived from the Greek meaning "eating of self". At first glance, that doesn't sound like a good thing... until we take a closer look. It actually means that after fasting for a certain amount of time, our body "eats" the weak/damaged cells for energy and recycles them to make new, healthy cells. This is extremely important because when autophagy is activated, it gets rid of the bad cells that have the potential to cause serious diseases down the line.

According to lifeapps.io, autophagy is an important process for cellular and tissue rejuvenation – it removes damaged cellular components including misfolded proteins. When your cells can't or don't initiate autophagy, bad things happen, including neurodegenerative diseases, which seem to come about as a result of the reduced autophagy that occurs during aging. Within 24 hours, (of fasting) your cells are increasingly recycling old components and breaking down misfolded proteins linked to Alzheimer's and other diseases.

Wow! Possible increased protection from neurogenerative diseases while achieving your weight-loss goals sound pretty awesome to me!

Reduced Inflammation

According to npr.org, inflammation can be a force for good, protecting against infection and injury. Acute inflammation occurs when you sprain your ankle or get a paper cut. It's part of the immune system's box of tricks to spark a defense and promote healing. But when that response is constantly triggered, over time it can damage the body instead of healing it. Chronic, low-level inflammation seems to play a role in a host of diseases, including type 2 diabetes, heart disease, Alzheimer's, cancer and even depression.

According to the Mayo Clinic, research suggests that intermittent fasting may be more beneficial than other diets for reducing inflammation and improving conditions associated with inflammation, such as:

- Alzheimer's disease

- Arthritis

- Asthma

- Multiple sclerosis

- Stroke

Reducing inflammation in our bodies is a must if we want to live long, healthy and vibrant lives. As opposed to a regular intermittent fasting routine, simply eating less does not have the same results in reducing inflammation.

In addition to all of the benefits that we've covered, medical professionals believe that there are countless more that we haven't discovered yet. With more research being conducted on intermittent fasting, science is constantly discovering more ways that it is beneficial to our bodies.

Weight Loss Benefits

In addition, the act of simply reducing fat and returning your body to a healthy weight carries many benefits with it, such as: decreased risk of diabetes; lowered blood pressure; improved cholesterol levels; decreased risk of heart disease; decreased risk of certain cancers; decreased risk of stroke; reduced back pain; decreased risk of osteoarthritis; decreased risk of developing sleep apnea; greater confidence; improved sex life; better sleep; elevated energy levels; decreased stress and better mood.

Saving Time and Money

It might sound crazy at first – but you will actually save time and money when you follow the One Meal A Day Diet!

Think about it – if you are only consuming one meal every day, it will save you time in the following areas:

- Deciding what you'll eat or drink

- Preparing the meals (or picking them up)

- Time spent consuming the meal

- Clean-up time afterwards

I understand this doesn't apply to everyone. Many of you, like me, still have to prepare food for your families. But for those who it does apply to, this will be a game-changer.

It might not sound like a lot of time, but it quickly adds up. If you didn't have to take all the steps listed above twice a day, you'll definitely have more time to dedicate to other things you'd like to accomplish. Even using a conservative estimate, you'll gain at least an hour back every single day. What could you do with an extra hour every day?

Another added bonus is that you'll save money when you follow this plan. For those of you with families that are still consuming the traditional three meals a day, this might not be evident right away. For those who only prepare your own meals (or for you and one other person), the difference will be substantial. This not only applies to the money you'll save at the grocery store, but you'll also save on dining out, take-out, snacks, etc.

Mental & Emotional Benefits

I personally believe that this is one of the most exciting changes that you'll experience. The difference that you'll see in your mental and emotional states will be mind-blowing. You won't have to talk yourself into feeling better – it will happen automatically and naturally. Two of my favorite benefits in this area are as follows:

You'll gain more self-confidence.

Not only because you're getting closer to your fat-loss goal, but because you'll be proving to yourself that you CAN be successful in this area of life. When we experience countless diet failures, it's easy to adopt an underlying attitude that conveys "I can't really do this." The doubt is always there. But when you start making strides and realize you can do it, your confidence will soar. An added benefit to this is that you'll start to notice this confidence spreading to other areas of your life.

You'll be free from a diet mindset.

When you no longer hold the mindset that you "can't have" certain foods or can only have a small amount, everything will change! When "forbidden" foods don't exist, it takes away all of their power. Personally, this was the single most powerful change in my mindset when I switched to intermittent fasting. After feeling like I was in a prison for countless years, I was finally free. The restrictions were gone and I could truly enjoy food once again without feeling guilty.

Fast and easy weight loss; transformed health; extra time and money; mental clarity and freedom? Sounds good to me! I hope you're getting excited. OMAD really is all these things and more.

Next, we'll have a look at what is happening inside the body to make this way of eating so simple and powerful. Let's move on to Chapter 3...

Chapter 3: What's Happening Inside My Body? The One Thing You Need to Know.

If you have an interest in discovering exactly what is happening inside the body when you practice intermittent fasting, there are countless resources available. Because 1) this is a quick-start guide and 2) I am not a doctor, I am going to boil this down to the single most important thing you should know about what is happening inside your body when you fast ...or when you break a fast.

On the other side of the coin, if you have absolutely no interest in the science behind what makes OMAD so powerful, I still believe that it is extremely important to know **WHY** you shouldn't have "just one bite" of pizza or "that one sip" of a delicious latte during your fasting hours. That *one* tiny bite or sip will set into motion metabolic processes that can throw off your entire fast.

Because there aren't many rules on OMAD, the ones that are in place *must* be followed to the letter. The first rule of OMAD is don't talk about OMAD. Just kidding. The first rule is to only consume foods and calorie-containing beverages during your eating window. Eating anything outside of that time will discount your fast and make it much less powerful.

If I'm having a weak moment or feeling hungry, I usually ask myself, "is it really worth a bite?" The answer is usually no. Again, there are times to be flexible such as family gatherings, being out with friends, a wedding or other celebrations, etc. But when it's a bite of a donut in the break room at work – skip it! You'll be happy you did. Here's why...

What Happens When We Eat? Extremely-Simplified Edition

When a relatively healthy person consumes calories (from food or a beverage), their blood sugar rises. The body responds by releasing insulin, the main hormone responsible for energy storage. Insulin takes the energy that has just been consumed and ushers it to the places it needs to go inside the body. Some of the energy is used immediately and some is saved for later use. A limited amount of this energy can be saved as sugar. This gives the body quick-access to energy for the near future. But once that limited short-term storage is filled, the body goes to work storing the rest as fat.

Insulin is our friend because 1) it takes the energy we've eaten and ushers it to the tissues and other areas of our bodies that need it, and 2) it helps to lower our circulating blood sugar levels, since it can be dangerous if they remain elevated. That being said, insulin can also be a friend that turns on us if we don't treat him well.

Listen up. Here's your main take-away for this chapter: **when insulin is present in the bloodstream, your body locks up your fat storage-units. No stored fat can be burned as long as insulin is present.**

That's it? Yep. That's it.

Well, of course that isn't really the entire story. Our bodies, which have been created in a miraculous fashion, go to work taking care of the countless processes that need to occur to keep us going. But, as far as what you need to take away from this chapter, that is it.

You only need to remember that insulin in the bloodstream interrupts your fast — no matter how small the amount of food. Again, it doesn't matter if it's one M&M or one sip of juice. The end result is that your body will release insulin. That is what we want to avoid during our fasting hours.

There is some controversy in the fasting community about whether weight loss comes about because there is a cap on the calories that can be consumed in a short period of time. Some people are convinced that this is just another way of restricting calories. Because I am not a medical professional, I cannot definitively answer that question. My opinion is that weight loss comes about as a combination of both. I believe that giving the body a chance to let the insulin levels drop (and therefore, make it easier to release fat from storage) in conjunction with an overall slight reduction in calories creates the perfect combination and the best environment for easy weight loss. From my experience, it is my opinion that 2/3 of the weight loss power in fasting comes from the decreased insulin levels and that 1/3 can be attributed to natural (not forced) calorie restriction.

According to dietdoctor.com, the body only really exists in two states – the fed state and the fasted state. Either we are storing food energy (insulin is in the bloodstream and we are increasing fat stores), or we are burning stored energy (no insulin is in the bloodstream and we are burning our fat stores).

When we eat from the time we get up till the time we go to bed, we never give our bodies the chance to be in fat-burning mode. This can only happen when we give it a complete rest, in the absence of any food or drinks that contain calories.

Our bodies are so used to being in the fed state, that we constantly need more to keep our energy up. Once you start giving your body the chance to rest and regularly enter the fasted state, you'll find that your body will be happy burning the stored fat.

When your body is in the fasted state, you'll find that you'll typically experience very little hunger. There is one caveat to this: you have to give your body the chance to adjust. Don't expect this adjustment to happen overnight. But it WILL happen. You will be amazed at how little hunger you'll experience during your fasts once your body adapts.

The reason you've felt ravenous after skipping a meal or two in the past is because your body wasn't used to entering the fasted state. This will quickly change. Plus, knowing that a beautiful and completely satisfying meal is coming soon will help you through hungry times in your adjustment period.

I hope this helps you to understand a fraction of what is going on inside your body when you're practicing intermittent fasting. If you want to know more, you can find countless resources online. For now, just remember this: insulin in your bloodstream = no fat burning. It's not worth the bite.

I'd like to give a small disclaimer and remind you that what is described above is what typically goes on inside a relatively healthy body. If you have diabetes, other health issues, or if you are on any medications (especially medications that regulate blood sugar), your body is most likely not responding in this way. It is extremely important to discuss this with your doctor and get their approval before embarking on this, or any other type of new eating regimen.

Next we'll dive in to every dieter's favorite questions: "What can I eat?" and "How much can I eat?" Join me in the next chapter!

Chapter 4: How Much Can I Eat & What Can I Eat?

When it comes to learning about a new eating plan, these are the questions that every dieter wants to know the answers to:

- How much am I allowed to eat? And,

- What can I eat on this plan?

The amazing news is that when you practice The One Meal A Day Diet plan, there are almost no restrictions on how much you are able to eat or what you can eat and still lose fat.

That being said, OMAD is **NOT** a license to binge once a day. As with everything, there is a balance.

Because every person is different, you'll need to discover what works for you and what doesn't. I wish I was able to give you clear-cut instructions in this section. But there is no one-size-fits-all approach. And isn't that really the beauty of it? You have the opportunity to design a plan that works for YOU. No one will be telling you what you can or can't consume. This is a wonderful thing because you can tailor the OMAD plan to your personal needs/preferences.

First, let's take a closer look at the amount of food you'll be consuming.

How Much Can I Eat?

The short answer is that you can have as much food as it takes for you to feel satisfied. Of course, this is not the entire answer.

Before we get into a few more details on this subject, I want to encourage you that you will not have to think too much about this. If you're new to fasting, your internal panic alarms might be sounding right about now. "What if I get so hungry that I eat everything in sight?" or "I won't be able to control myself!" I promise you, that within a couple of weeks, this will cease to be one of your worries. It might sound completely foreign right now, but once you are used to this new rhythm of eating, you will not want to eat as much as you have in the past. That's right. And this is coming from a former binge-eater!

I don't have the scientific reason behind this phenomenon – but I do know that it takes a much smaller amount of food for me to feel full. Give yourself some time to adjust. The first 2-3 weeks might not reflect this. But be kind to yourself. Expect that it will take some time to fully adjust and for your hunger to dissipate (more on hunger later).

I wanted to start with that encouragement to save you from worrying about managing the amount of food that you will eat when fasting. OMAD is a way of eating that will *free* you from all of the over-thinking and micro-managing of food. Your body will tell you when it is done eating. You'll have to be patient with yourself in this area too. It will take some time to re-learn what the correct amount is for you.

I have spent many times feeling stuffed and overly-full after my OMAD meal. Other times, I tried to restrict myself (which was a mistake), and I'd feel hunger sooner than I'd like to. As you start to pay attention and become more in-tune with your "feeling full" cues, this will be easier to navigate.

Another factor that plays in to how much you'll be able to consume and still lose fat is your current weight. When I started, I needed to lose almost 100 pounds (about 45 kilos). Obviously, someone needing to lose 20 pounds (about 9 kilos) would not be able to consume the same amount of food as I could at that point. Although you'll have to do a bit of self-discovery and see what works for you, (again) I don't want you to get too hung up on this, because I honestly believe it will become obvious and self-regulating – even for those who have a history of extremely poor eating behaviors, like I did.

What Can I Eat?

Again, the short answer is: you *can* eat anything that you would like (during your eating window). But because everyone has different likes/dislikes, sensitivities, allergies, preferences, cultures, etc. What you choose to consume will vary from person to person.

That being said, my suggestion is to start your meal with wholesome foods in their natural state. Some examples of these types of foods are non-processed meats, fish, eggs, nuts, seeds, fruits, vegetables, etc. If you choose to abstain from consuming meat, starting with a protein source will serve you well.

The reason it is best to begin your meal with these types of foods is that they offer much more nutritional value than processed foods. For your body to perform at the optimum level and for you to feel good, you need these nutrients! Plus, it is easier to get them in at the beginning of the meal. The odds are that you won't squeeze them in at the end. Then you can move on to any treats or desserts that you'd like to incorporate.

For example, I usually eat my foods in this order: meat, salad or vegetable and then bread and/or dessert. I save my treats until later in the meal, since I'm less likely to overeat on meat or salad.

When I'm ready for my treat, I enjoy it freely. *No guilt allowed*. Please do the same. My hope for you is that you will learn to fully and thoroughly enjoy your food once again. Instead of carrying around guilt over what you "should" or "shouldn't" eat, you can re-learn a good relationship with food. The best part is that this will come naturally over time. You won't have to force it.

As I briefly mentioned in the last chapter, although calories do play a role in your weight loss, you don't have to be overly concerned with them... and *please do not* start counting calories (unless you enjoy that type of torture). OMAD is designed to free you from the shackles that have held you back in the past. Simply eat in your "eating window"; give it some time and everything else will fall into place. That being said, if you have a very small amount of weight to lose, you might not be able to eat as much as you'd like to. Although I still wouldn't suggest counting calories, you might want to limit treats and/or breads to a few times a week, instead of having them every day. Follow what your body is telling you.

What Can I Consume During My Fast?

In order to set yourself up to have the most success with The One Meal A Day Diet, you should only consume the following during a fast:

•   Water (filtered or sparkling, no additives). Add lemon, if desired.

- Black coffee

- Unsweetened tea

That's it. That might seem scary at first glance. But if you think of all the amazing benefits that IF can provide: the easy weight loss and being able to eat almost anything you want during your eating window – this is totally worth it!

If you're wavering, review Chapter 3 and remember that **insulin in the bloodstream = no fat being released**. Drink some water, tea or coffee and tell yourself that your next delicious meal is right around the corner.

Next we'll cover how to get started with OMAD and how you can choose to ease in or jump in like a cannonball. Join me in the next chapter.

Chapter 5: Getting Started with The One Meal A Day Diet

Like everything in life, there are varying opinions on the best way to start intermittent fasting, especially the OMAD plan. I will once again tell you that there is no "right" way, so you should do what is most comfortable to you.

Some people ease into the practice and others simply jump right in. I am a "let's-jump-in" type of person. So when I started, I simply decided on an eating window and one day I restricted myself to only eating during that time and I didn't stop.

If that sounds crazy and scary to you, no worries. You can ease into it. Here are a couple of suggestions on how you can do that.

Skip A Meal

Does only skipping breakfast sound less intimidating? Or perhaps eating breakfast and lunch while skipping dinner sounds better to you. Either way, pick a meal and start regularly skipping it. The key is consistency. The more you do it, the more your body will get used to this new eating pattern. Once you're used to it, you only have to skip one more meal to get to OMAD.

You can stay with skipping one meal for days, weeks or months. Whatever it takes for you to feel comfortable moving to the next level.

Shrinking Your Eating Window

Let's say you are currently eating from 7:00 a.m. when you have breakfast until you have a snack at around 9:00 p.m. That means that you are currently eating in a 14-hour eating window. You can start by shrinking your eating window by an hour per week (or whatever rate is comfortable for you). You'll keep shrinking the window until you achieve the 23:1 OMAD window.

Tip: Once you reach a 4-hour eating window, you're basically already where you need to be. It's hard to fit in more than one truly large/satisfying meal in less than 4 hours. As I sit writing this, I ate my OMAD meal 3 hours ago and I still feel comfortably full. Plus, you'll be sleeping 6-8 hours a night, which will take up a large part of the fast. You'll get there sooner than you think you can.

You WILL Experience Hunger

I wish I could say that you won't. But you will experience hunger. I want you to be prepared ahead of time, so you will have realistic expectations. In our culture we're not used to being hungry. We typically grab something to quench it as soon as it arises.

The good news is that it *will lessen* over time. It is usually the most pronounced in the first week or so while your body is adjusting. As time goes on, you will feel less and less hunger. There are days that I feel no hunger whatsoever. This is a typical response in people who practice IF. That being said, there are days that I do still feel hungry. Here are a few tips that can help you overcome the hungry times:

• Drink water, tea or black coffee.

• Remember that hunger comes in waves. Just wait it out. It might seem overwhelming... and then it will simply disappear.

• Do something to distract yourself (work, play, etc.)

• Tell yourself that your next wonderful meal is just around the corner. It's worth the wait.

• Change what hunger means to you. Instead of it signifying lack or deprivation, tell yourself that you are BURNING FAT from your fat stores.

Losing weight (especially if you've carried extra weight for a long time) can be a battle in the mind even more than a physical battle. If we can make these simple changes in our thinking, it can completely transform our outlook on the process. If we get stuck thinking thoughts such as: "Poor me! I'm deprived. Look at what my family is eating. I want some. This isn't fair!" it's easy to ride that slippery slope down to a bad place. But if we start reminding ourselves that soon we'll be able to enjoy a delicious and satisfying meal, while the fat falls off... it will be easier to stick to only eating in our eating window.

Instead of thinking "I *have to* stay on my plan." switch it to "I *get to* follow a simple plan in which I can eat whatever I desire until I'm satisfied, while losing fat! How awesome is that?"

If you eat outside of your window, be kind to yourself. Just get right back on. We all go off plan sometimes. But the good news is that is extremely easy to get back on the OMAD plan. Most dieters, including me in the past, tend to have an "the diet starts Monday" attitude. Once we fall off, we eat everything in sight until it's time to "get back on". With OMAD, there are no forbidden foods, so it takes this destructive attitude out of the equation. So what if you ate in a 4-hour window one day? Just get back to your 1-hour window tomorrow. Easy. You'll be pleasantly surprised at how easy it is to eat (and be successful) in this way. I can't wait for you to discover this for yourself.

Chapter 6: Do I Have to Exercise to Have Success?

You may be asking, "do I have to exercise in order to have success with OMAD?" Once again, I'll give you a short version of the answer as well as a longer explanation.

The short answer is no. You do not have to work out in order to see amazing fat loss results with OMAD. That being said, there are countless benefits that are associated with exercising and being active. Therefore, I highly encourage you to have some activity in your day (if you don't already).

It seems as though many people have a negative attitude towards exercise. I think this is derived from a collective attitude of "I *should* be more active." It's that *"should"* that makes it sound like a chore, so we interpret and internalize it in that manner. But what if we looked at being active in a new light? Remember back to when you were a child. Most children love to run around, ride their bikes, play sports, skateboard, play with pets, play tag, you name it! As we get older, it turns into a "should" rather than a "I get to". As a kid, you'd think "I get to play outside!" as an adult, we think "I have to exercise".

What if we could get a bit of that enjoyment back into our lives? Try taking a walk, playing a sport you used to enjoy or biking around the park. Try to switch this back to being an "I get to" activity.

Any of these activities can be fun and done at a leisurely pace. As a society it seems that we've made everything *extreme*. The "go big or go home" mentality has driven many of us to stay home! When it's a fun and enjoyable activity rather than an extreme energy-drain, it becomes something that we can look forward to, instead of something we can't stand doing. Anything we dislike doing will not be sustainable in the long run. That's the bottom line.

One last encouragement to you regarding exercise... when your body is in the fasted state, the only place it can pull energy from is your fat stores! Therefore, when you do any activity in the fasted state, it burns the fat right off your body. Instead of having to burn through the sugar in your bloodstream and "short-term" storage areas, it targets the stubborn fat you've been storing on your body. If that isn't motivation to get out and move, I don't know what is!

If you've enjoyed this book and feel like you've benefited from the information, would you please leave me a quick review? I would truly appreciate it and you will be helping others find this information as well. I read every review and I would love to hear your feedback!

Conclusion

Thank you so much for letting me lead you through this quick-start guide of The One Meal A Day Diet! I hope that you're excited to get started. I wish you all the success in the world. I pray that you will discover and claim all of these amazing benefits in your own life. Don't let this information simply remain as words on a page - get out there and give it a try! It might be challenging at first. But if you make it through 2 days, you've made it through the hardest part. Don't give up! Keep going. Because it will only get easier from there. I can't wait for you to see the results for yourself.

If you've enjoyed this book and feel like you've benefited from the information, would you please leave me a quick review? I would truly appreciate it and you will be helping others find this information as well.

Part 2

Introduction

The One Meal a Day (OMAD) Diet is a weight loss method based on intermittent fasting, meal frequency, and meal timing. It is a way to lose fat and keep it off, while eating whatever you want.

This is not a fad diet, nor is it a temporary weight loss solution. A short term diet is unhealthy and will increase your weight when you stop the diet, indeed many dieters have experienced a yo-yo effect on their weight. They do not lose enough weight to be satisfied, and end up giving up their diet.

The issue is that these diets do not address the root cause of weight loss, which is to manage the circadian rhythm. This is done by timing exercise, meals and sleep; two of which we will look at in this book.

The reason the OMAD diet works is because it is a lifestyle, and one that that works for the long term because it is based in science. If you can follow the plan you will improve your health, energy, and well being. You do not have to count calories, worry about what you can or cannot eat, and mostly you do not have to feel guilty for cheat days.

In this book we will explore the OMAD diet and its benefits, as well as how you can use it in your own daily life. We will also look at the risks, especially diabetes which is on the rise in America. We will consider how the OMAD diet works with keto, another popular diet these days, as well veganism which is a philosophy as well as a dietary choice. Adding these food restrictive diets to OMAD can work, and may provide additional benefits to your diet. However, the dietary requirements of OMAD and keto, or OMAD and veganism, will place additional demands on your body as well.Lastly, I will share some testimonials of people who have tried and succeeded with the OMAD diet.

Where possible I will make reference to scientific studies or medical publications as the OMAD diet, Intermittent Fasting, and Time Restricted Feeding have emerged from the halls of medical laboratories and research desks.

Chapter 1: The Obesity Epidemic

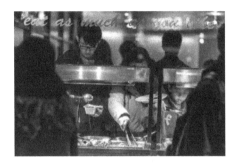

In most cultures it is common to eat three meals a day. Also, we think nothing of having snacks even if it is just one square of chocolate, one piece of candy, or a mouthful of potato chips. According to the National Health and Nutrition Examination Survey 1999-2000, about 80% of Americans eat four or five times per day.

Is it any wonder why obesity has been called an epidemic in modern society?

In 1960 9.7% of Americans were obese, and this has been a rising trend since then. In 2012 about 34.9% of adults were obese. Today it is estimated that the number of obese or overweight people in America is around 70%. Diabetes, which is a common ailment of the obese has increased seven fold in the same period. Every year it is estimated that almost 400,000 deaths each year are due to obesity related illnesses.

Aside from the frequency that we eat, there are many other factors that expert believe have contributed to this epidemic.

So why are we getting more and more obese?

1. Food technology has improved. Vacuum packing, preservatives, and microwaves have made access to food more easily available.

2. Stressful lifestyle. America is one of the most overworked countries in the world with more than 65% of people working more than 40 hours per week. As stress increases, we turn to eating as a means of venting steam.

3. Lack of exercise. As we spend more and more time in front of a screen, we spend less time on physical activities. A sedentary lifestyle can lead to obesity. The Department of Health & Human Services (HSS) has estimated that less than 5% of adults participate in 30 minutes of physical activities each day.

What Causes Weight Gain?

While there are many causes such as genetics, food availability, lack of exercise, and the abundance of sugar in our diets the main cause of weight gain, however, has been found to be due to a disruption in circadian rhythm.

The circadian rhythm is a biological process that happens in a 24 hours cycle and responds mainly to light. Eating and sleeping are two examples of this, but it also controls our body's cycle of fat burning and fat storing among others.

Because of the circadian rhythms in our bodies there will be variations in our hormone and enzyme levels which affects how the food we eat are processed. These feeding signals then are the main cues that your circadian rhythm triggers your metabolic, behavioral, and psychological pathways that influence the overall health of your body. Ultimately, how well synchronized your circadian clock is working with your schedule and how well it is synchronized with the day/night cycle determines your overall health.

When you skip meals, or eat late at night it increases the likelihood of weight gain because it can raise blood sugar and cholesterol levels in your body and affect your appetite. Your metabolism is also affected, which can affect your digestion, which leads to you feeling lethargic, getting hunger cravings, and accumulating fat.

A high calorie diet, lack of sleep, improper eating habits, in sufficient exercise, and too much or too little light can disrupt your circadian rhythm.

Why Diets Fail at Helping You Lose Weight

Diets usually focus on the foods that you can or cannot eat in order to maintain a calorie deficit. The idea is that if your body burns more energy than it takes in, you will lose weight. However, this works against your body as it leads you to take food that is low in nutritional value. If you are not satisfied with your meal, it leaves you hungry.

Research has also found that reducing food intake can increase your risk of binge eating as it prompts your brain to develop cravings. The more you deny yourself food, the more you are likely to end up wanting to eat.

Majority of people are also likely to regain the weight that they have lost while on a diet, maybe even gaining more weight than they originally had. It is common for many people to stop dieting once they lose weight, only to regain the weight, and then go on another diet. This is known as yo-yo dieting.

This is because most diets do not address the core issue of weight gain which is managing the body's circadian rhythm. And as we learned in the previous section, regulating the body's circadian rhythm with exercise, proper meals, and sufficient sleep is vital to helping the body lose weight.

Why OMAD Helps You Lose Weight

While it is often called a diet, as you will learn in the upcoming chapters, OMAD is actually a lifestyle. The principles of the OMAD diet are based on the many scientific studies done over the years, putting together the best of what works in losing weight, as well as keeping off the weight that you lose.

The Journal of the Academy of Nutrition and Dietetics published a study 2015 on "Intermittent Fasting and Human Metabolic Health" found that people who fast have lower cholesterol and blood sugar levels, improved gut microbiota, and a more active metabolism. The OMAD diet gives your body 23 hours to get the benefits of fasting.

The logic behind this ties back to ancient times when humans needed to hunt or forage for food. Our ancestors did not have late night pizza joints, grocery stores, or vending machines, they would only eat during the day and fast at night.

When you fast, it forces your body to adapt to the stress. Your gut in particular has better function and gets less inflamed because it is not constantly working to digest food. This makes your body more resilient against diseases such as heart disease, inflammation, and even cancer. Fasting has also been proven to improve sleep and reduce obesity.

The timing and consistency of your meal is key for the OMAD diet. It works because it makes our bodies adapt to a lack of glucose by using a more metabolically efficient state to work with your circadian rhythm. Your body will only have a small one hour window to get food so it does not accumulate too many calories that are stored as fat. Then, your body has 23 hours to work through the fat stores in your body.

It provides a simple and straightforward method that can achieve a permanent weight loss, there are many testimonials on the OMAD diet in the last chapter that you will read about later on.

Chapter 2: Starting on the OMAD Diet

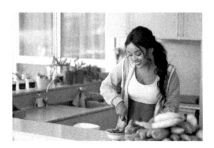

While eating one meal a day may sound simple at first, there is a recommended approach to this diet. Like any other diet, the beginning of the switch in eating habits will require conscious effort to maintain, and you will need to build on this consistently in order to achieve long term success. When you are consistent in your daily eating habits, the diet starts to take effect and help you achieve the weight loss that you have set out for yourself.

The basis of the OMAD diet is the rule of 4 "Ones".

The Rule of 4 "Ones"

The easiest way to understand the OMAD diet is to look at the rule of 4 Ones. In essence, this means you should have:

1.   One Hour
2.   One Meal
3.   One Plate
4.   One Beverage

This rule helps you to maintain the discipline and have a structure to your diet. Many people have found this method to work best for weight loss, as well as maintaining a long term healthy lifestyle. So how do you follow the Rule of 4 Ones?

One Hour

When starting the one meal a day diet, you need to choose a four hour window to eat. This can be any four hours you want, but make sure it will best fit into your schedule as it would be best to stay consistent with the eating window.

Once you have chosen your four hour window, you should allow yourself one hour for your meal so you have sufficient time to enjoy your food which can include a beverage of your choice. When the hour is up, there should be no more calorie intake until the next eating window.

When choosing your eating window, it might take some time to figure out how to choose the best one to fit your situation, but maintaining a structure will make all the difference in your weight loss journey.

One Meal

Each day, you will have a 4 hour eating window but you should only give yourself 1 hour in those 4 hours to eat. In that one hour, you will have only one meal.

In the OMAD diet, there should be no small meals, or cheat hours where you can eat snacks or junk food.

The only exception to this are for protein shakes taken post workout. If you do workout, these protein shakes are necessary to fuel your body with protein.

One Plate

Since you are restricted to one meal, it may be tempting to pile on whatever you want in your one hour window. When you are eating your one meal, it's important to understand what is going on your plate, and ensure that there is a balance of nutrients, proteins, and carbohydrates.

It is recommended to incorporate a serving of vegetables, carbohydrates (potatoes, rice, or bread), protein and fats (from meats), and a serving of fruits. The caloric intake for most people during OMAD is around 1,500 Kcal.

An average sized plate could actually hold two servings of meals so it is important that you make an informed choice of what goes onto your plate and not overeat during your one meal.

One Beverage

During your meal, you should allow yourself to have one beverage of your choice. This can be anything you crave, from beer, to a soda, or anything else you want. This serves as a perk me up to boost your mood. The OMAD diet is not about depriving yourself, it is just a structured way to approach your food and drink intake.

Taking a drink with a caloric count can also help you to get your calories required for the day, but you should keep yourself to one serving.

Apart from this, you should continue to hydrate yourself by drinking water throughout the day. You do not have to limit your intake of water. Tea and coffee can also be drunk at any time, as it may help to suppress your hunger.

What to Expect When Starting OMAD

When starting out on OMAD diets, the first thing most people experience is hunger so you are not alone. This is most likely an issue of body conditioning that you will have to battle the first few weeks. You may not actually be hungry, but because you have been eating several times a day, your body has been conditioned to expect food every few hours.

While this will vary from person to person, a "fasting headache" is common for the first few weeks at least. This is triggered by a combination of low blood sugar, dehydration, and possibly lack of sleep. The trick is to stay hydrated throughout your fast.

The brain is 75% water and is very sensitive to dehydration, and produced histamines to ration and conserve water when faced with a shortage. It is these histamines that cause headaches as well as fatigues; they are a signal that we need drink more water. Keep in mind that this discomfort will end once your body gets used to your new eating schedule and the lack of intermittent snacks throughout the day.

Keeping yourself busy with work or distracting yourself by immersing yourself in other activities will help you think less about food. Staying away from the kitchen or the pantry will also help as you will not be constantly seeing and smelling food to whet your appetite when it is not your meal time.

Once your mind has been disciplined to eat only meal a day, your body will adjust eventually.

Starting OMAD

When starting out with the OMAD Diet, there are a few things you need to keep in mind to make your journey easier and keep you motivated and disciplined throughout. While it may seem easy to just eat less frequently, we all have our own schedules, priorities, willpower, and physiologies to consider.

1. Set Goals

Before you start on the OMAD diet, you should have a clear goal in mind. Generally, people who go on diets are either looking to:

1.   Lose weight
2.   Maintain weight
3.   Improve their health

If you are dieting for weight loss or maintenance, you should set a goal you would like to achieve. Then set up some sort of system to track how you are doing, as well as record your habits. Remember that you should be burning fat as a source of energy.

If you are dieting for health, then you might want to get your doctor to run a series of tests for you on your cholesterol levels, your triglycerides (liver function), and your fasting blood sugar at the very least. You can use these as a marker to ensure that you take balanced meals and get the nutrition your body needs.

Mark any accomplishments you have, no matter how small. When you start to see small successes such as sticking to one meal a day, or losing a single pound off the scales it will be much easier to follow through.

As with any diet, your body needs time to adjust so having a timeline will make it easier for you to stay focused on your goal.

2. Prepare Yourself

Few people who jump into a diet actually succeed in their goals. It is recommended that you take a couple of weeks to ease yourself into the diet. Make sure you are mentally prepared, and that this can work for you and your lifestyle before committing fully.

This is also a good chance to consult with your doctor or nutritionist; you should only start your diet once you get the all clear from them.

3. Start Cutting Your Daily Meals

If you are currently eating three or more meals a day you can start by cutting snacks out of your diet. Then you can try to time your meals by having 4 meals, 4 hours apart, slowly cutting the meals and the hours between meals by one each time. Eventually you will be at one meal a day.

If you are really hungry, it is recommended that you take a bowl of bone broth. It is packed with minerals as well as amino acids that helps with extended fasting.

4. Give Yourself Some Slack

OMAD means "One Meal A Day", but it is common for people to mix things up and do this semi regularly. Maybe they do OMAD on days that they do not go to the gym, or they choose to only skip one meal instead of two each day. As you will see in a later chapter, there are many people who practice this diet in different ways.

It is also common for some people to expand their eating window to 4 hours or 8 hours instead of 1 hour. That is known as intermittent fasting, and there are many people that will testify to its effectiveness at weight loss as well.

"Cheat days" are pretty common in diets, but they do set you off course from your goal. In OMAD, a "cheat day" would be one where you have more than one meal since there are no restrictions on the kinds of food you can or cannot take.

If you need a "cheat day" to maintain your sanity, it is a personal preference. It can be hard to say no to a beer with the guys, or a cocktail on a girl's night out just because it happens outside your one hour window. Still, be sure to regulate your fat and sugar intake and get back to eating one meal the next day.

Being consistent is key in any diet, including OMAD. Just be sure that you are getting enough food, and you stick to the 4 "Ones" Rule.

Risks of OMAD

Every diet requires discipline, but OMAD more so than others. Deciding to embark on an OMAD Diet may also require you to decide in advance how much you are willing to commit to it. OMAD Diets are extremely effective, only if it is properly followed and maintained.

Only by following the 4 "Ones" Rule, and properly training your mind and body to overcome hunger pangs will you succeed. Remember that it is possible to achieve your weight loss goals that you set out for yourself, but it all depends on your dedication to the diet.

That being said, there are also some risks to OMAD that you would have to be aware of.

OMAD is ideal for people who need to maintain or lose weight, so if you are bodybuilding or trying to gain muscle mass, it may benefit you to eat more regularly as your requirements are probably more than you should intake in a single sitting.

There are also serious risks for people with preexisting medical conditions such as diabetes. Diabetics suffer from low blood sugar, also known as hypoglycemia, and need to eat meals regularly throughout the day to avoid any serious side effects.

Pregnancy may also affect your decision to go OMAD. As pregnant women in their second and third trimesters (basically after 3 months of pregnancy) need to consume extra calories. While medical research in this area is still inconclusive, it is not recommended by most doctors to fast while pregnant as it can lead to complications like low birth weight of the child.

If you have suffered from eating disorders, it is also not recommended to try OMAD. It is not worth choosing your mental health over your diet. Every time you fast, you are actively helping your eating disorder to take over your life.

In any case it is advisable to consult a doctor before beginning an OMAD Diet.

Eating one meal a day can also have physical side effects such as weakness, exhaustion, and a lack of focus. Physical symptoms such as extreme hunger, weakness, fatigue, and being unable to concentrate may also appear in some people.

Hydration is important in dealing with most of these, but it is also important to consider your own personality. If you are unable to stick with the plan of the 4 "Ones" Rule and go full OMAD, you might want to consider other diets.

You Should Not Fast If...

You should avoid fasting if:

- You are pregnant or breastfeeding
- You have a history of an eating disorder
- You have a history of a sleeping disoder
- You are underweight

Also you must consult a doctor first if:
- You have a long-term medical condition (e.g. cancer, diabetes, ulcerative colitis, epilepsy, anemia, liver, kidney or lung disease).
- You have a condition that affects your immune system.
- You are on medication.

The Key to Going OMAD Successfully

Since successful weight loss with the OMAD diet requires that you restrict your intake of calories if you are to lose weight and realize some of the benefits that are associated with the diet; having some insight on what the macronutrients are is therefore vital.

Here is an overview of the macronutrients that the body needs in order to function well.

Protein: When working out your muscles essentially break down and your body requires protein for building muscles and recovering from your training. While it is commonly found in meat and dairy, protein can also be found in nuts and legumes. The rule of thumb for athletes and bodybuilders is to have 1 gram of protein for every pound of bodyweight. Each gram of protein is equal to 4 calories.

Carbohydrates: Carbohydrates aka carbs are the body's main source of energy, and are comprised of fiber, starch, and sugar.

Simple carbohydrates are generally absorbed into the bloodstream faster and cause a spike in blood sugar. Sugar is a simple carbohydrate.

Complex carbohydrates take longer to digest and are absorbed into the bloodstream slowly. They do not cause a spike in blood sugar. Fiber and starch are complex carbohydrates.

Each gram of carbohydrate is equivalent to 4 calories and the sources of calories are grain, bread, pasta, rice, potatoes and sugar.

Fats: Fats are also very important for optimal body health and it gives your body a store of energy. Fat is also needed to keep your skin and hair healthy, as well as to absorb certain fat-soluble vitamins. There are three types of fats: saturated fats, unsaturated fats, and trans fat.

Saturated fats can raise your LDL (bad cholesterol), and too much of it can put you at risk of serious medical issues like heart attack and stroke. Foods that are high in saturated fat are dairy and animal products.

Unsaturated fats can lower your LDL. They are found mainly in vegetable oil such as olive oil and canola oil.

Trans fats are the result of vegetable oil hardening and can both raise your LDL (bad cholesterol) and lower your HDL (good cholesterol). Avoid these where ever possible. Trans fats can be found in margarine, microwave popcorn, frozen pizza, and some cake frosting.

Caloric maintenance: Caloric maintenance is the number of calories that your body requires each day in order to be in a state where it does not lose or gain weight. Caloric gain tends to vary from person to person with factors such as age, gender, muscle mass, and lifestyle needing to be taken into consideration.

If you are to lose weight then the caloric intake should be lower than what your body expends in a day. Each pound of bodyweight is approximately 3,500 calories. To find out your recommended caloric intake, you can use an online calorie calculator.

Chapter 3: What You Must Know About the OMAD Diet

The Benefits of OMAD

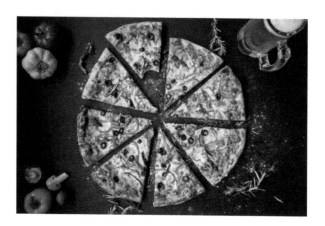

Regardless of why you have chosen to adopt the OMAD diet, here are a number of benefits you will realize almost instantly. Most of this you will experience after a short time after adopting this diet.

Weight Loss That Sticks

The obvious benefit of OMAD is the weight loss that comes from sticking to the diet. By limiting yourself to one meal, one plate, and one beverage in one hour (the 4 "Ones" Rule), you are limiting your caloric intake. Snacks and other junk food have a large amount of calories that we are not aware of, and cutting them out helps us to lose weight and keep it off.

Most people will cut back up to 1,000 calories a day by staying away from the vending machine, potato chips, and chocolate. This can quickly shed up to a pound a week if maintained.

While other diets result in losing water weight resulting in dehydration, the OMAD Diet encourages you to constantly hydrate to stave off hunger headaches and fatigue. This means that any weight loss is truly fat loss rather than just dehydration.

If you manage to stick to the diet plan and consistently exercise discipline in what and when you eat, it becomes a lifestyle change that sticks with you for good.

Burn Fat

When on the OMAD diet, you ideally want to be burning fat as an energy source and the fasting period of your diet is a great way for burning body fat. When you are sleeping the body naturally gets into a fasted state where it automatically switches to a fat burning mode, and fasting prolong this natural fasting state. When you wake up and begin eating, your body produces insulin and starts to use the carbohydrates you consume as energy instead of fat.

Cholesterol Control

It is a common misconception that decreasing dietary cholesterol may reduce blood cholesterol levels, but the cholesterol in our blood is generated by the liver. A 2012 study on cholesterol by AIM-HIGH Investigators showed that LDL (bad cholesterol) is reduced when fasting by up to 25%.

This is alongside other benefits such as reduced body rate and decreased waist size, as well as preserving HDL (good cholesterol) levels. This happens because the body switches from burning sugar, to burning our fat reserves when fasting.

Blood Pressure Control

By eating less junk food and snacks, you are cutting out a lot of sodium (salt) from your food intake. This has been backed up by many researches.

A study published in Nutrition and Healthy Aging has found that fasting has reduced blood pressure by up to 7% in a number of individuals who participated in clinical studies. While the sample size is small, it does show promise.

Coupled with the weight loss benefits, and improved cholesterol, a reduction in blood pressure all contributes to a reduction in the risk of heart disease.

Blood Sugar Control

By not snacking outside of the eating window, you are also cutting back on sugar. This has the effect of lowering blood sugar, which is the concentration of glucose in the bloodstream. Blood sugar levels are also a result of carbohydrates such as rice, bread, and potatoes.

When we eat, insulin brings these sugars to our cells that are stored as fat.

When we do not snack between meals insulin levels will drop and fat cells will start to release the sugar that they have stored. Therefore, by cutting down on our blood sugar, insulin levels are reduced and our bodies will start to burn fat.

Improved Digestive System

Since you are eating only one meal a day, your digestive system isn't as overworked as before. If you reduce highly processed and fatty foods, digestive issues will be reduced even further.

If you have irritable bowels or other gastrointestinal issues, the OMAD diet can help because you will not constantly be trying to process food in your gut. Gradually, you will feel better after meals.

Improved Immune System

There are many reports of people getting sick less often, and having more energy with OMAD due to an improved diet. Many researchers have found that fasting may also reduce the risk of chronic diseases, including heart diseases.

When we stop eating and focus on resting, this reduces the stress on our internal systems. The energy we use to digest our food can instead be used for boosting our immune systems, our cognition, and other brain and body functions.

Drinking water while the body is fasting also allows our digestive system to flush out any micro organisms resulting in a better regulated immune system which means that we are healthier on the OMAD diet.

Supercharge Your Brain

Dr Mark Mattson, a Neurology Professor at John Hopkins University has found that fasting increases the growth and development of brain cells and nerve tissues.

Additionally, fasting has also shown to reduce inflammation in the brain which can lead to Alzheimer's and other neurodegenerative disorders.

This is in line with what other people who fast have reported in terms of increased concentration, and better memory. This also results in being more mentally stable and alert during daily tasks.

A More Positive Relationship With Food

The OMAD diet when followed, can change a person's psychological approach to food. Because you are allowed to eat whatever you want in your eating window, food is no longer viewed as negative.

People on the OMAD diet have a healthier relationship with food, enjoying whatever they want instead of having secret "taboo" foods that they avoid only to binge on.

Counter intuitively, binge eating is also less likely to occur since the diet is about consistency. With the variety of food open to dieters, people are less likely to restrict themselves for long periods only to go wild on what they want to eat.

The OMAD diet is not about restriction, but rather about eating a regular amount at a regular time. People have reported that they are less likely to want to eat anything and everything, but have a better relationship with food through this diet.

Part of having a healthier approach to food is also enjoying food more. People on OMAD have shared that they appreciate the taste of food more. They savor each bite that they take, and are able to enjoy exploring new spices and cooking styles in their diet.

Better Productivity

Usually, our bodies rely on the food we eat to give us energy by converting carbohydrates to sugar and then breaking it down. When we deprive ourselves of food for a long period like 23 hours, our blood sugar levels drop, and as a result insulin levels drop as well.

Our bodies then learn to look for an alternative source of energy, and turns to the fat we store.

Since we only eat once a day, our metabolism changes. When using fat instead of food as energy, fat needs to be slowly digested and sent to the liver for processing. This process happens steadily over time, and unlike eating does not have spikes in our blood sugar, or our metabolism.

With the use of coffee and tea, you can still use caffeine as a source of energy, as well as to trick your stomach into thinking you have eaten even though you have not.

A Lifestyle Change

Although it is called a "diet, OMAD is actually a lifestyle change and brings with it many benefits.

Discipline is a huge factor in succeeding with the OMAD diet, and it can be difficult at times to deal with the discomfort and the hunger, especially in the initial stages. This is a long term thing, to maintain the self discipline not just for a day, or a week, but for life.

To be successful, you need to learn to transition to one meal for the rest of your life.

When you managed to do this, take a moment to realize that you have managed to follow through with this diet and maintain the self discipline required to stick to the diet. The same self discipline that helped you to do this can be applied to other areas of your life as well. You can learn to change your habits, and the mindset that helped you succeed in your diet can be just as applicable.

From there you will not only feel better about yourself and experience all of the benefits listed above, you will also eliminate the possibility of relapsing into poor eating habits.

Guidelines for Going OMAD

When starting out on any diet, there are many do's and don'ts, the same goes for OMAD diets. While fasting has been around for ages in many different forms and for many different reasons, it has gained in popularity in recent times among dieters, athletes, and gym goers. This is due to their desire to improve their health, lose excess fat, and shed the pounds.

While it sounds convenient, there are many fasting plans which can make the diet confusing. In this chapter we will look at the guidelines for starting an OMAD diet.

Stay Hydrated

The OMAD diet allows for the consumption of water, tea, and coffee as long as they are unsweetened. Water is especially encouraged as proper hydration can stave off headaches and fatigue, even when you are not doing OMAD.

Branch-Chain Amino Acids (BCAA) and protein shakes are also recommended for bodybuilders, gym goers, and athletes especially after training.

Working Out

People claim that fasting improves their workout due to its beneficial effects on testosterone and growth hormones. Fasting can boost your performance in the gym, as well as your overall strength, so working out with weights or high-intensity exercise can improve the effects of the OMAD diet.

Eat Balanced Meals

What you put into your body determines how efficiently it works so be sure to eat a clean, balanced meal. Make healthy choices by including items from every food group.

The recommendation is to base meals on starchy food like potatoes, bread, rice, and pasta. Multi-grain or wheatmeal options are a better choice as they are more complex carbohydrates and take longer to digest.

Include protein such as meat, fish, eggs, or beans (tofu counts). Protein is used to build and repair tissues, including bones, cartilage, skin, blood, and especially muscles.

Fruit and vegetables are a vital source of vitamins and minerals. It is recommended to have at least 2 servings of each. Fruit and vegetables are also a good source of fiber that will keep your gut and digestive system healthy.

Do Not Overindulge

While the OMAD diet allows you to eat whatever you want, as long as it is in your eating window, it does not mean that you should binge on junk food like cookies, potato chips, chocolates and cake.

Making healthy food choices is the key to making this diet work, although you can (and some people argue should) indulge in a bacon cheeseburger or a pizza if that is your fancy as long as it is not too often. Remember that fasting for hours will not balance out the fat and sugar from a binge.

Listen to Your Body

If you feel dizzy, weak, or sick stop dieting and eat something.

When starting out, many people experience fatigue and headaches, but with proper hydration, sufficient sleep, and a bit of time your body should overcome these symptoms.

Hopefully you got your doctor's permission to go on this diet, and if these symptoms persist more than a week you should consult your doctor again. Fasting will affect your blood sugar which can lead to complications if you have other medical conditions (even if you are unaware of them).

Please diet responsibly.

Your Weight Will Fluctuate

Depletion of salt in your body can affect your weight by up to 4 pounds in a day depending on your food intake.

Eating starchy foods that are high in carbohydrates, or high salt content can cause water to retain in your body thus leading to a weight gain. Likewise, going to the toilet, and exercise can lead to a temporary weight loss.

The thing is to track your weight at a consistent time each day, and watch the trend over the next few weeks. You should find that the long term results would be a downward trend. So there is no need to get worried if your weight fluctuates during the day, especially after meals.

Side Effects of the OMAD Diet

In this chapter, we will look at the side effects that people who start the OMAD diet commonly face. Most of this are a result of fasting for long periods, and people commonly encounter these in the first few weeks of fasting which everyone agrees is the toughest phase of any diet but especially the OMAD diet.

All of these symptoms may sound scary, but remember that it should last only a week. Most people report the same thing as well. However, remember that the OMAD diet is not for everyone.

If you experience difficulty in performing your job or your family responsibilities, or if you feel discomfort, dizziness, or faint you may want to consider breaking the fast early.

Remember to be kind to yourself, and also remember that your brain and your body are going through changes.

Hunger

Your body is used to eating three times a day, and maybe with snacks in between, and it has learned to expect food at certain times. The hormone known as ghrelin is responsible for making us feel hunger, and has been found to peak around meal times.

When you begin fasting, you can expect ghrelin levels to continue to peak around these times, especially the first week but eventually it will pass. Some people have reported that during their meal windows, they don't even feel hungry.

When starting a fast, drinking water will help to combat the hunger. Some nutritionists explain that the hunger may be dehydration or boredom as eating three times a day is a habit that we have been conditioned with all our lives. Drinking unsweetened coffee and tea may also help with hunger similar to drinking water.

Cravings

Food is an integral part of our lives. We use meal times to bond with our friends and loved ones, so outside our fasting window it is natural for us to think about eating and cravings will kick in.

It will also be likely that since our bodies are without food for a long period, it is common to want something sweet, or unhealthy junk food for that quick hit of glucose in our blood stream. The good news is that with the OMAD diet you can eat whatever you want, as long as it is during your meal time.

The trick is to distract yourself with other tasks and not think about food. Keep yourself busy, or go for a walk to keep your mind busy. Whatever it takes, it will need willpower to push through especially in the early stages of your diet.

Headaches

With the OMAD diet, headaches and fatigue are common especially when starting out. Dehydration is a major factor in this, so drinking lots of water will help with this as well.

Headaches can also be caused by low blood sugar levels or by the stress hormones released by your brain while fasting. Before your body adapts to your new eating schedule, try to remain as stress-free as possible.

Fatigue

Since your body is not getting energy from multiple meals and snacks, you can expect to feel fatigue more easily than before. It is normal to feel your energy levels lower during the initial phase, so try to keep your daily activities as relaxed as possible.

If you do exercise, you may want to consider going easy. Walk instead of run, or you may consider having an extra (smaller) meal or a protein shake on days you work out. This should not be taken as a free pass for a second meal or junk food however.

Lastly, getting extra sleep or taking a nap may help with this as well.

Feeling Cold

When blood sugar decreases, this makes us more sensitive to the cold. When deprived of food, our bodies goes into what is known as adipose tissue blood flow. This means that blood goes to our fat stores, to move the fat to our muscles where it can be used as fuel.

Be sure to prepare for this by wearing thicker clothing, sitting near a radiator, or turning down the air conditioning.

Emotions

When fasting, it is common for unexpected emotions to come up from time to time. Without knowing it, a lot of us turn to food to suppress emotions. That's why "comfort food" is a thing. So when we cannot suppress emotions through food we have to deal with them in other ways.

Feeling irritable is also pretty common as you are dealing with other side effects. Learning to keep your calm and being mindful of your actions would help, as will focusing on activities that you enjoy.

Overeating

People tend to overeat when they are new to the OMAD diet. This can be due to the fact that they are unaware of the calories they need, or a fear that they will not have enough food to last them until the next meal.

It may also be a case of feeling extremely hungry by the time your eating window comes around that you end up eating really fast, and take in extra portions.

Plan out your meals ahead of time, and try to stick to it.

Under Eating

This one is more for people who have already successfully been on the diet for a while. Whether due to a lack of time, or a worry about calories remember that your body needs to get its energy. Take your time and eat until you are full, and ensure that your meal is balanced.

Remember the Rule of Four "Ones"? You are allotted one plate of food, and you should stick with it.

Foods You Should Be Eating

While there are no restrictions with regard to the type of food you can eat when on OMAD, you will see a better result if you eat a balanced meal and make healthy choices. Taking the time to plan the food you eat, or at least give a little thought to your meals, will reap benefits for your health and metabolism.

Here are a list of things you should consider:

Have enough calories in your meal. If you do not consume enough calories during your eating window it will very likely lead to you feeling weak and fatigued. It is likely then that you would have to break your fast early.

Reduce carbohydrates. When you take a large amount of carbs your blood sugar will spike and your body will release large amounts of insulin. However, while carbohydrates make you feel full it digests faster than proteins, leaving you hungrier. You may also want to consider taking complex carbs like brown rice, wholemeal bread, oatmeal, and sweet potatoes among others. These take longer to digest and will provide your body with energy for a longer period.

High fiber vegetables. Broccoli, sprouts, cauliflower, and leafy vegetables are full of fiber which is consider a complex carbohydrate. These can be very filling and help you through your fasting window and also have been proven to lower cholesterol.

Have fish once a week. Eight ounces of fish will help you get a lot of healthy fats and proteins. Since your body has a limited amount of food each day, having a nutritious food packed with nutrients and vitamins is recommended.

Eggs for more protein. Each egg contains 6 grams of protein, which helps to keep you full for longer. While you should be taking other forms of protein, consider the boost that an egg will give you as well.

Have a serving of fruits. Fruits are a great source of vitamin and minerals, and are also a source of fiber. Blueberries, citrus fruit (like oranges and lemons), cranberries and strawberries also contain phytochemicals that are believed to have added health benefits.

Probiotics for your gut. Probiotics comes mainly from fermented foods and improve your digestive health. This is especially important when fasting as you want to ensure that your digestive system is not over stressed. Foods like yogurt, tempeh, kimchi, and miso have high amounts of probiotics that your body needs.

Drink lots of water. As we will cover in the next chapter, water is essential to your health and well-being. When you are sufficiently hydrated, your body can operate at peak efficiency and help your metabolism as well. Dehydration especially when fasting can lead to all sorts of complications.

Chapter 4: The Importance of Water

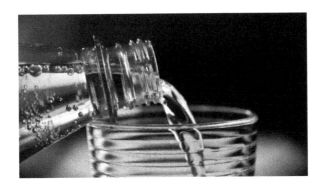

Staying hydrated is important at all times, but when fasting it is even more important. Since our bodies are up to 65 percent water, and our brains are 75 percent water, failing to stay hydrated could damage our bodies.

In this chapter, we will look at the importance of water on the OMAD diet. Why we should be hydrating? How much should we drink? And also, what should we drink?

Why Drink Water?

Your body will not function properly without adequate water, as it is needed to carry out its everyday processes. In fact, your body needs pure water more than it needs daily food, as you can go without food for much longer than you can go without water.

Here are some of the benefits of staying hydrated.

Burn Fat

A 2016 study published in Frontiers in Nutrition has found that increased water intake is linked with weight loss. So staying hydrated can help you to achieve and maintain a healthy weight. This is due to a process called lipolysis, and it is triggered when water molecules interact with triglycerides.

Control Hunger

Very often, when we feel hungry, we are actually dehydrated. Drinking water can also help to suppress the appetite; it makes feel full and tells your brain to stop eating.

A researcher at Virginia Tech by the name of Dr Brenda Davy has found that drinking two glasses of water before a meal led to quicker and more significant weight loss. This can result in eating up to 75 fewer calories at each meal, which can add up over time.

Boost Metabolism

Metabolism is how your body processes food and water to give you energy. When your body is unable to use the food that you have put in, it starts to store the excess food as fat. By increasing your body's metabolism, you decrease your fat storage.

Drinking one glass of water can increase metabolism by up to 30 percent, and on the other hand being dehydrated will reduce metabolism as well. This is due to the fact that drinking water helps to increase the number of calories we burn by digesting the water.

Stay Feeling Energized

When fasting, energy is very important as we would not want to feel lethargic and fatigued. When we are sufficiently hydrated, our cells are primed to convert food and body fat into energy. When we are dehydrated the functions of our body will slow down as they are not able to function properly.

How Much Water to Drink When Fasting?

The 8 x 8 rule which suggests 8 ounces of water 8 times a day has been debunked as a myth in a 2002 study published in PubMed by Valtin H.

So what is the recommended amount of water we should drink then, and how would fasting change that?

The answer is "it depends on you". Different people have different hydration needs as it depends on their lifestyle and activities. When we are thirsty, it is a signal that our water intake is insufficient.

Simply put, there are 3 simple rules to follow with drinking water:

1.   When you feel thirsty, drink!
2.   When you stop feeling thirsty, stop.
3.   When you exercise, or are expecting hot weather/environments compensate for the lost fluids.

When fasting for extended periods of time, you may want to drink a little more to combat hunger and help your body metabolize fat. You should be drinking more water than what you are usually drinking when not fasting, and it should make your first few weeks less uncomfortable.

A Note on Overhydration

While dehydration is often talked about, overhydration can happen when we drink too much water and can be just as dangerous.

Overhydration happens when our bodies have more fluid than our kidneys can remove. A quick way to know our hydration needs is to look at the color of our urine. Too dark and it means we are dehydrated, too clear shows overhydration, and if it is a light yellow we are good.

Generally speaking, around half a gallon of water or liquids a day should be fine for most people. However, if you are feeling constantly thirsty, you should consult your doctor as it may be a sign of other medical issues that you should be aware of.

What Should We Drink?

Most food such as meat, fish, fruits, and vegetables all contain some amount of water. Plain water then is not the only source that contributes to our required daily water intake. In this section we look at the options of beverages we have while on the OMAD diet's fasting window.

Remember that during your eating window, you should allow yourself one beverage of your choice. That can be anything you crave or desire. But when outside your eating window, your options are a lot more limited.

Drinks you should consider

Mineral Water - Your body can absorb some of the minerals in water, and mineral water gives your body more minerals which is not a bad thing.

Green Tea - It is rich in antioxidants which can help prevent inflammation, cancer, and other ailments. Green tea has also been known to promote weight loss by thermogenically increasing your metabolism.

Herbal tea - Common in Asian cultures, it blends the benefits of herbs with benefits of hydrating yourself with a drink. Herbal teas may have medicinal properties, but remember to avoid any sweetened versions.

Coffee - Coffee can help you hydrate, as the diuretic effect is very weak and caffeine can provide you an energy boost as well. However, you should remember to avoid taking any sugar or milk with your coffee.

Chapter 5: Understanding Psychological Hunger

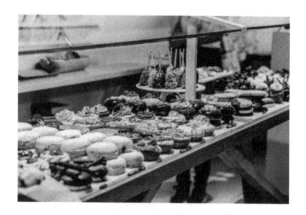

An evolutionary biologist by the name of Daniel Lieberman has found that humans evolved to crave sugar for energy when food was scarce. This is a hunger that ignites a desire to eat either out of habit, or because you see your favorite food available.

Studies done at Columbia and Rockefeller Universities have found that appetite is controlled by a hormone called ghrelin, which is released at regular times during the day. Furthermore, it was found to peak around mealtimes.

In this day and age there is no shortage of food especially if you are living in a developed country.

Therefore, when we eat it may be for pleasure or to counter boredom, in addition to other reasons. Hunger then has an underlying psychological cause and we might feel hungry even when we do not actually need food.

When fasting on the OMAD diet, remember that you are trying to lose weight by burning fat and eating less. You should learn to distinguish the difference between psychological hunger, and a physical hunger.

Physical Hunger vs. Psychological Hunger

Physical hunger starts with a physical feeling of emptiness in your stomach and is usually accompanied by rumbling. This happens gradually, and intensifies when postponed. When physical hunger occurs, any type of food will satisfy you.

Psychological hunger on the other hand, happens suddenly and has no physical symptoms. It is simply the desire to eat, and could be a craving for a specific type of food (usually something sweet).

Address and managing psychological hunger then is important as ignoring it will just cause it to grow until it is too difficult to put aside. What usually happens then is that you go on a binge and put on the pounds that you have already lost, and end up feeling guilty about the episode.

Once we realize this then it's clear that all it takes is a little bit of unwiring until our body adjusts to an OMAD diet.

Here is a quick comparison between the two to help you understand the difference between physical and psychological hunger better.

Physical Hunger		Psychological Hunger
Happens gradually		Happens suddenly
No specific cravings, any type of food will do	Vs.	Craving specific food (usually sweets)
Eat until you are full		Eat more than usual, feel bloated
Feel satisfied after eating		Feel guilty after eating

Dealing with Psychological Hunger

To control psychological hunger, the first step is to understand what triggers your psychological hunger. Everyone of us will have different triggers, and different reasons why we desire certain foods. We need to identify what causes the cravings we have, before we can deal with it.

Psychological hunger has nothing to do with our physical well-being, but our mental state; usually this has something to do with our emotions. Psychological hunger is sometimes referred to as emotional eating or stress eating.

This usually surfaces when we feel the need to compensate for something that has shaken our emotional state. For example, if you have just been through an argument with your significant other you may reach for a tub of ice cream. Or after a long grueling week at work, you crave a plate of fried chicken and gravy. There are always triggers to psychological hunger, and you need to identify those so you can develop a strategy to prevent those triggers from overwhelming you, or removing them altogether.

These emotional triggers may sometimes be signals that we are in a toxic environment be it a job, relationship, or lifestyle. These emotional needs resulting from stress, anger, depression, and boredom can easily cause your diet to go off track and if it happens too often you may need to seek the help of a trained professional as these issues can be too complex to unravel and address on your own.

Removing temptation is also a lot easier than trying to resist it. If you have food and snacks easily available, it will be much more difficult to avoid snacking when you feel overwhelmed, bored, or hungry. Stay away from the kitchen, and avoid buying cookies, chips, or other snack food when you go to the supermarket. If you have to prepare your snack you may feel less inclined to eat.

Chapter 6: OMAD and Diabetes - Is It Safe?

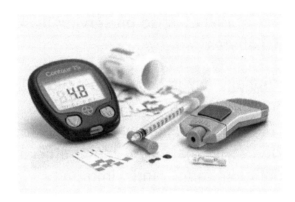

The OMAD diet is popular with people suffering from diabetes to lose weight and lower their blood sugar, but it does contain some risks. Critics say that the spike in blood sugar from eating one meal is unhealthy, while others point to the fact that weight and fat loss actually helps to regulate insulin levels.

While there are many opinions on OMAD and diabetes, the best way to approach this would be to look at the science done on the topic.

Studies on Diabetes and Fasting

The journal Cell Death & Disease did a study on autophagy, the consumption of the body's own tissue which occurs during fasting, in August 2017 that discovered fasting helped to preserve beta cells in mice with diabetes. The beta cell loss and insulin resistance are markers of diabetes, so preserving beta cells helps to control diabetes.

When autophagy occurs, the cells in your body create membranes that seek out dead, diseased, and worn-out cells and use the resulting molecules for energy or regeneration. This makes us more efficient and can control inflammation and immunity, and some scientists believe that it may be the key to slowing down the aging process.

A study published by the World Journal of Diabetes in April 2017 observed the health markers of a small number of adults with type 2 diabetes has shown that fasting for 18 to 20 hours a day can lead to better levels of blood glucose control. This not only improved fasting glucose levels and weight, but also the after meal blood sugar levels.

The potential of this study is that short term fasting maybe a safe and dietary method which can lead to improvements in the body's insulin sensitivity.

The first study was done on mice, which are mammals and share a large portion of their DNA with humans.

However, it is no guarantee that the same methods would have similar benefit in us.

The second study was done on humans, but the criticism is that the sample size is rather small, containing 9 males and 1 female for a grand total of 10 participants. This may not be representative of all people as a whole as it was not a randomized and controlled study.

However, I have confidence that studies on fasting and eating one meal a day for diabetics are only in the early stages. It is only a matter of time before a more in-depth study is done with more conclusive results.

The Risks of OMAD for Diabetics

The main criticism of OMAD and any other extended fasting diet for diabetics is that blood sugar needs to be kept at a stable level.

Skipping meals not only leads to poor blood sugar control, but also leads to issues like fatigue, low energy, and interference with medication. Extreme hunger from fasting may also lead to poor diet, which will have a negative effect on your blood sugar. Needless to say, overeating during mealtimes will also cause weight gain which will work against any efforts in controlling diabetes.

While losing weight can be beneficial for diabetics as it increases the body's sensitivity to insulin, gaining weight will have the opposite effect. This can lead to an increased risk for diabetes complications.

What you eat during your one hour window on the OMAD diet can also negatively affect your blood sugar. Eating too much carbohydrates and sugars will raise your blood sugar levels and cause erratic readings throughout the day.

When talking about diabetes, high blood sugar is not the only issue. Hypoglycemia, low blood sugar, is another concern that diabetics have to watch out for. BMJ Global Health published a study in September 2016 showed that 10 percent of people who fasted regularly experienced hypoglycemia, and certain medication may increase the risk of this.

Hypoglycemia in diabetics can be life threatening, so while 10 per cent might not seem like a lot, the consequences are severe.

Lastly, ketoacidosis is a complication where diabetics cannot produce enough insulin in their bodies. When the body does not have enough carbohydrates to process during fasting the body overproduces ketones.

Too much ketones could result in damaged kidneys and brain swelling. Diabetic ketoacidosis may even lead to a diabetic coma or death.

Whether you have diabetes or not, reducing meals and changing your diet can cause nutritional deficiencies. A lack of carbohydrates will affect blood sugar and ketones, a lack of protein will risk a loss in muscle mass. Experts have therefore strongly recommend that medication and lifestyle should be adjusted prior to fasting, and these strategies should only be planned and implemented with the help of a doctor.

How to Go OMAD with Diabetes

The first step before switching to an OMAD diet is to consult your doctor. Discuss with him or her a diet and medication plan, as well as to ensure you clear your food choices with them. Diabetics on insulin need to be especially careful as they are at greater risk of hypoglycemia, which may lead to severe consequences.

If you do get the all clear from your doctor to try OMAD, it will help you to stick with the diet if you join an online community, social network, or at least have a friend doing it with you.

Decide on a plan that you can stick to long term. While OMAD means one meal a day, there are many people who use this diet only for the short term, or on alternate days, or just several times a week. The idea here is to find something that works for you.

Be prepared for the side effects, but know when to quit. We have discussed the side effects in an earlier chapter. Headaches, fatigue, cramps, are all common ailments that people suffer from OMAD, but if you are throwing up or feel very unwell consider stopping and consulting with your doctor. Remember to diet responsibly and listen to your body.

Have a balanced meal every time. Just because you're on OMAD does not mean that you should eat anything and everything you want, especially because diabetics need to consider the effect of food on their body and the blood sugar levels. A healthy diet will help keep your weight under control, and your blood sugar levels steady.

Go for whole, unprocessed food like multi-grain options, and include vegetables, protein and healthy fats in each meal. Hydration is also very important to keep headaches and fatigue at bay.

Lastly, manage your expectations. OMAD is not for everyone and even for those people who have made it work may have failed several times. If you quit, remember that failure is not final you just need to adjust your strategy and you should consult with your doctor again.

Instead of OMAD, maybe a less extreme diet may work better for you, and may be a healthier, happier way for you to lose weight.

The Bottom Line for Diabetics

The research on this is split on both sides at the moment. While there certainly are benefits to OMAD and fasting, there are also severe risks involved.

While the OMAD diet may help you lose weight, which can help you better control diabetes, it is important to consult with your doctor. The main thing is to have a diet that is sustainable and safe for you, and your doctor will be able to make an informed decision especially if you do a blood test for diabetic health markers.

Chapter 7: Working Out on OMAD

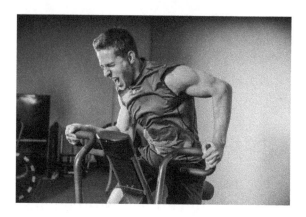

Exercise is crucial to improve your physical and mental health and reduce the risk of chronic disease. Even when you are on a diet, exercise should still be a part of your routine.

However, when in a fasted state and on the OMAD diet, you have to take special consideration to your energy levels and the demands exercising will place on your body.

Exercising in a Fasted State

According to a study on meal timing and physical activity in 2017 done by the University of Bath, has suggested that exercising on an empty stomach has a number of health and fitness benefits. Eating before exercise has shown to reduce the long term effects of exercise on our lipid, insulin, and blood sugar.

Exercise is more effective in a fasted state for two reasons.

Firstly, fasting can trigger a dramatic rise in human growth hormone (HGH), also known as "the fitness hormone." HGH is secreted when we sleep, and is believed to be related to anti-aging since it typically decreases as we get older.

It is also known to increase our muscle growth and improve exercise performance. After fasting for three days HGH levels can increase by up to 300 percent, and after a week it can increase by up to 1,250%.

This works because fasting helps you to burn body fat, which increases HGH production, and it lowers insulin levels which research has shown to disrupt HGH production.

Secondly, our bodies sympathetic nervous system is activated by both the exercise and the lack of food. The combination of fasting and exercising forces our bodies to breakdown fat and glycogen for energy, meaning we are burning fat more effectively in a fasted state.

When exercising in a fasted state, our bodies burns off the stored sugar and then starts to work on the fat we have stored, converting it into ketones for fuel.

There are many studies that have shown that the additional fat loss by exercising in a fasted state is increased by up to 20 percent. When not fasted, insulin is increased in our body, and higher insulin levels are linked with a slow-down of fat burning metabolism by the same amount of approximately 20 percent.

This basically means that exercising on an empty stomach makes our bodies more efficient at using fat rather than sugar as fuel.

When to Work Out on OMAD

The short answer is to work out before you eat your meal.

While common wisdom is to work out in the morning because of the reasons covered above. However, if you are on the OMAD diet, you are in a fasted state until you have your meal so working out in the morning may mean a stretch of a few hours until your meal.

This can be challenging if the period between the end of your exercise and the start of your eating window is too long. Waiting for the eating window to open may be difficult enough for some people, and having to wait for it after working out only makes it much tougher.

Remember that your body needs to refuel after an intense work out.

Instead, I would suggest you consider scheduling your workout two hours or two and a half hours before your meal. Try to keep an hour between the end of your workout and the start of your meal as this is when experts believe is the post-exercise anabolic window.

The theory is that consuming nutrients an hour after exercise is supposed to be more effective at rebuilding muscle tissue and restoring energy.

Remember that the OMAD diet is about consistency, so plan your routine to ensure that it works best for you. We all have our own commitments and priorities, and therefore our schedules are very different.

If you have to schedule your exercise much earlier or later than your meal time, you should consider breaking your fast.

Have a protein shake, or protein bar before your exercise if necessary but eating after your workout is highly recommended. Eating after a workout stimulates muscle protein synthesis and improves the recovery from your work out session. It also helps to enhance your performance during your next work out.

Also, remember to stay hydrated. Water is essential to replenishing and revitalizing your body.

BCAAs and OMAD

First let's get one thing clear about Branched Chain Amino Acids (BCAA): They break your fast.

BCAAs are supplements that contain amino acids, which are the building blocks of protein. There are 9 amino acids in total, but the main ones that BCAAs contain are Valine, Leucine, and Isolecuine.

BCAAs have a caloric value of 6 Cal per gram, and will trigger an insulin response in our bodies because they contain proteins. Since fasting is meant to keep your insulin levels low, taking BCAAs will break your fast.

Whey, casein protein shakes, eggs, beef, chicken, and fish all naturally contain BCAA, and if eating any of those would break your fast, it is the same with taking a BCAA supplement.

Casein Protein Powder and OMAD

Similar to BCAAs, casein will also break your fast.

Casein is a slow digesting dairy protein consisting of 80% milk protein. This means that it feeds your cells with amino acids over a long period of time.

A lesser known fact about casein is that it helps to synthesize protein, even when your body might be breaking down its own muscles. This happens when fasting, and it makes casein beneficial for an OMAD diet as the slower digestive process keeps the amino acids in your body longer.

In addition to the above, there are some more benefits found in research on casein:
- *Antibacterial and immune benefits:* casein may provide antibacterial and immune benefits as well as reduce high blood pressure.
- *Fat loss:* fat loss is improved by three times when on casein
- *Reduction in free radicals:* peptides in casein protein powder may have antioxidant effects.
- *Triglyceride levels:* casein reduced triglyceride levels after a meal by 22%.

Your Diet when Working Out

If you're on the OMAD diet and want to build muscle bulk, a high amount of protein is necessary for muscle synthesis. Your muscles are broken down during exercise and repair themselves throughout the day for growth, and protein is necessary for this process.

Studies have shown that the ratio of protein intake to bodyweight is roughly 0.13% to 0.18%. Meaning that you need about 0.2 - 0.3 ounces of protein for every pound you weigh although other factors such as the intensity and frequency of your workout, your age, and your gender can affect this.

Bodybuilders have a similar rule of thumb where they take 1 gram of protein per pound of their body weight. Some even take up to 1.5 grams per pound of body weight when trying to lose fat.

Aside from proteins, carbohydrates are an important part of our diet. It is recommended that we eat whole-grain cereals (with low-fat or skim milk), whole-wheat toast, low-fat or fat-free yogurt, whole grain pasta, brown rice, fruits, and vegetables when working out on the OMAD diet.

Sugars and grains are also carbohydrates, but should be avoided as much as possible along with processed food. These foods cause cravings as well as our blood sugar to spike severely which overworks our body's digestive system. After the "sugar rush" also comes a crash in blood sugar which brings about hunger and the craving for more food.

Last Words on Exercise and OMAD

Remember that our bodies are different, and we all adjust to routines differently. The important thing is that we are consistent with our diet, our eating window, and our workout routine as the OMAD diet is a lifestyle.

When making any changes to habits, introduce them one at a time and give it some time to take effect and show results otherwise it will lead to frustration.

Lastly, remember to hydrate yourself before and after your work outs. I know I have said it several times in this book, but the effects of dehydration can be severe. Exercising while dehydrated has been linked to kidney failure, seizures, and even death.

Chapter 8: The OMAD Keto Diet

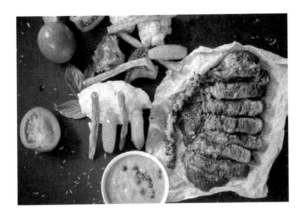

The OMAD diet has been often paired with the popular ketogenic or keto diet. Some people have even gone as far as calling it a match made in heaven.

What is the keto diet? What makes OMAD and keto go so well together? We'll cover all these questions in this chapter.

What is the Ketogenic Diet?

The ketogenic or keto diet is about getting your body to enter a state known as Ketosis, that is when your body burns fat and protein instead of carbohydrates.

When the body digests carbohydrates and sugars introduced into the body, insulin is produced in the body. Insulin is meant to help process this and when the carbohydrates have burned, it will result in a crash in energy levels. This causes cravings for food again, which may result in people overeating.

While sugars may provide a source of quick energy, it comes at a price to your body.

Fats and protein on the other hand are very dense and will provide you with consistent energy throughout the day until they are digested. If your diet is filled with healthy fats and proteins, you can expect to feel full and energetic throughout the day.

However, Ketosis only takes effect if your body has next to no carbohydrates in it.

Getting Your Body into Ketosis

As mentioned, ketosis is when the body burns fat and protein instead of carbohydrates.

So the obvious way and one most often suggested is to reduce your intake of carbohydrates. When you reduce your carb intake, glycogen stores are reduced which in turn lowers the insulin in your body. This forces the fatty acids in your body to be released from the fat stored in your body, and your liver can then convert these acids into ketones.

Another way to get your body into ketosis is to increase your physical activity as exercise depletes glycogen stores as well. When glycogen stores are low, the liver produces ketones to metabolize the fatty acids stored in your fat.

A third way, and one most common for people on the OMAD diet, is by fasting. When the carbohydrates in our bodies are burned up as energy, and no food intake happens our bodies are then forced to go into ketosis. In fact many people go into a state of mild ketosis between their dinner and breakfast the next day. The OMAD diet just prolongs this by keeping the fast for a longer period.

The last method is by using certain foods. Food like avocado, cheese, yogurt, eggs, fatty fish (salmon, trout, and tuna), olive oil, and coconut oil it is possible to boost ketone levels. Coconut oil contains medium-chain triglycerides and has been suggested that it may be one of the best ways to increase ketone levels.

Note that doing this may work against weight loss if you consume too many calories.

If you choose to go keto with OMAD, you should test your ketone levels regularly. Because our bodies are all different, we will react differently to exercise, food, and supplements. You want to ensure that your body is in ketosis, and your liver function and triglycerides are healthy.

Bringing Keto to OMAD

The extreme fasting window of at least 20 hours when on the OMAD diet will often trigger ketosis. This is true even if you have eaten carbohydrates, since they will be used up as energy in a few hours. After that, your body will begin to go into ketosis and burn fatty acids.

Eating one meal a day combined with the keto diet is possible and many do it with success; the keto diet and OMAD diet have a lot in common which encourages people to use the two diets together.

On the OMAD diet, the body is more likely to suffer from a severe sugar crash a few hours after your feeding window. Because your body will use sugar as an energy source quickly, it will leave you feeling hungry even if you eat a lot of starchy foods. This can be easily countered by adding fat and protein to your diet which is the purpose of keto.

Once your body burns through sugars and carbohydrates, it will turn to your stores of natural body fat. As a result, it won't need the sugars in carbohydrates to stay active and healthy. This change dramatically decreases your urge to eat and makes getting through fasting even easier.

However, before you decide to do this there are certain things that you need to be aware of.

Firstly, this is a major dietary change and your body will need to be able to adapt to it. Paired with the OMAD diet which has its own adaptations needed, you might want to consider introducing these changes one at a time especially because of the dietary restrictions of the keto diet.

This restricted diet alone is a challenge for many people to manage, as the adjustment period is complicated by the cravings you will experience for carbohydrates when starting out. While these will go away after a few days, your body will crave sugary carbohydrates because it is so used to using them to fuel your body with energy from sugar.

Secondly, there are misconceptions that keto and OMAD is an unhealthy dietary combination that can cause harm to a person's body. That is only true if you do not follow a professional's advice when changing your diet.

There are many professionals that believe the keto diet should only be used under supervision as it can damage muscle and lead to complications. Therefore you should consult your doctor as well before taking this step. They can help you to adjust your diet and ensure that this is the right step to achieve your dieting goals.

While keto and OMAD are perfectly safe when correctly implemented, it is possible that you end up with insufficient food or create a nutritional imbalance without a professional guiding you.

Keto and OMAD have a unique series of benefits worth exploring. If you are interested in trying either of these diet styles out, it is worth knowing why they work so well together and how keto can help with any intermittent fasting method.

One of the most difficult parts about the OMAD diet is the feeling of hunger most people experience before, during, and after your feeding window.While other people may have difficulty just getting through the 20 hour fasting period. The ketogenic diet helps with this by making you feel fuller than you normally would, and also by preventing a sugar crash.

Benefits of Keto and OMAD for Diets

As we can see in the previous section, there are many similarities between the OMAD diet and the keto diet. In this section, we will look at the benefits of practicing both OMAD and keto diets.

1. Improved Ketosis

The main goal of the keto diet is to put your body in a state of ketosis. This occurs only when there are no sugars or carbohydrates in your body to burn as fuel. Eating all of your food in one meal instead of spreading it out throughout the day will cause your body to turn to your fat stores more easily.

This change makes your body enter body-fat-burning ketosis more rapidly and will provide you with a boost of energy. Even better, it will help you slim down and lose weight more quickly than eating your meals spread out through the day.

2. No More Food Comas

When we eat too much carbohydrates, our bodies start to use energy to digest all the food we have eaten. Our bodies are lethargic from this process, and we naturally feel sleepy.

However, when on OMAD and keto, you will be able to think more clearly and be more alert. Your body will perform more efficiently with less carbohydrates and sugars, by burning fat and protein instead.

3. Improved Metabolism

When starving, our metabolism naturally slows down to conserve energy and get the most of the resources still within our bodies. It is natural then to assume that when on OMAD and deprived of carbohydrates on keto, our bodies will be on starvation mode.

However, that is not true.

Starvation mode only happens when our caloric intake is under 1,2000 calories per day over to course of a week. Fasting for long periods causes the body's metabolism to increase as it adjusts to the new schedule, as well as to make sure it digests food when it is available.

When ketosis kicks in during the fasting period, metabolism can increase even further.

4. More Effective Exercise

People on OMAD and keto have reported that their body's digestion and ability to stay active improves, making them healthier and more energetic.

However, remember to take a protein shake or bar before exercise as it will provide energy for your work out. It will also reduce fatigue and muscle strain. Also keep in mind that you should break your fast no more than two hours after exercise, again to provide fuel for your body.

5. Reduced Insulin Levels

For people who suffer from an imbalance in insulin levels, such as diabetics, fasting is can be used as a means of treatment. This is especially true in the case of combining keto and OMAD.

When limiting the intake of carbohydrates, insulin becomes less necessary for day-to-day activities. Lower levels of insulin can also help burn more fat since insulin stops the body from burning fat by converting sugar into energy.

6. Better Liver Functions

Combining OMAD and keto has a positive effect on your liver. The liver is a store of fat and glucose, but excessive amounts can cause damage to your liver over several years.

When on OMAD and keto together, the fat and glucose stored in your liver will decrease as it is used up. While there will still be some fat stored in your liver, it will be less fatty than before, and liver functions will be improved.

If you have liver diseases, it can be managed by OMAD and keto together.

Risks of OMAD and Keto Diets

As with any diet, there are potential side effects to be aware of and you should discuss these with your doctor. Adjusting to the demands of OMAD and keto may work for some, while others are just not able to integrate it into their lifestyles.

It helps to be aware of them beforehand, and if you choose to combine OMAD and keto, do so with full preparation.

1. Eating Disorders Can Get Out of Hand

If you have a history of eating disorders, OMAD or keto alone may cause complications. Combining the both of them may even make it worse or it may cause some people to develop an eating disorder that they did not previously have.

While issues like anorexia or bulimia may be the first eating disorders to come to mind when thinking about diets, binge eating should also be discussed.

Remember that before trying out any diet, you should have a positive body image and be in good mental and physical health. Otherwise, it is possible for to get obsessed with your diet and suffer from emotional issues.

2. Health Issues

Constipation - The keto diet very often causes people to suffer from severe constipation, and introducing OMAD will complicate this further.

It is necessary to eat food with a lot of fiber, such as leafy vegetables, as well as to take fiber supplements. There have been cases of people who had bowel obstructions while on this diet, which can cause a lot of pain and discomfort. Severe cases of bowel obstruction can damage your intestines, or even lead to death.

Stressed Thyroid - The storing of higher levels of fat and protein may cause stress to the thyroid or adrenal glands.

The higher levels of stress are common to those who lead busy lifestyles, work longer hours, or have eating disorders. While stress hormones must exist for proper thyroid function, it is further increased as your body adjusts to the new eating schedule and diet.

3. Food Intolerance

With the focus on fats and proteins, it is possible to develop intolerances, or worsen them on the OMAD keto diet.

Usually this happens by overeating a single type of food, such as cheese or dairy being the most common culprits. There are also instances of people developing intolerances to carbohydrates as the body gets unused to eating carbs.

Food for Keto Diets

The keto focuses on eliminating nearly all carbohydrates in your diet and focusing on protein and fats. This is done to trick your body into entering the ketosis state.

The foods that are recommended for the keto diet are:

- Grass-fed meat (beef, lamb, goat, and venison)
- Fish and seafood
- Pork
- Poultry (chicken, duck goose)
- Eggs (of all types)
- Butter, gelatin, and ghee
- Saturated fat
- Non-starchy vegetables (bok choy, spinach, chives, celery stalk, asparagus, cucumber)
- Avocados
- Water
- Black coffee
- Mayonnaise
- Mustard
- Pesto
- Pickles

You should also occasionally eat some root vegetables, sea vegetables, full-fat dairy, high-fat seeds, and zero-carb sweeteners. The amazing thing about the keto diet is that you can eat as many calories as you want and you will still lose weight.

However, the OMAD diet focuses on limiting your food intake to a specific eating window during the day to limit the total number of calories in a day.

Chapter 9: The OMAD Vegan Diet

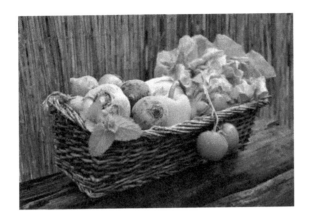

Veganism has been gaining in popularity, with a surge in late 2015 as people are more interested in how it could improve their health as well as their lives. There are also a growing number of people who adopt a vegan diet for the welfare of animals.

If you are among this crowd, it is possible to be vegan, and be on an OMAD diet. In this chapter we take a look at what veganism is, what benefits it has, and how to eat an OMAD vegan diet.

The Vegan Philosophy

Veganism is more than just a dietary restriction followed by millions of people around the world, it is a philosophy that rejects the commodity status of animals.

The diet of a vegan centers around not eating the meat as well as the product of animals (such as milk or eggs), it also extends to by products as well such as stock, flavoring, food coloring, or anything else that may be made by or from an animal.

However, as mentioned veganism is more than just a dietary restriction. It also extends to the use of animal products and by products in other parts of their lives. There are vegans who would on principle, avoid wearing any leather or fur products or even cosmetics that have been tested on animals.

In general, vegans are against anything that may cause harm to animals. However, there is a range of diverse viewpoints and beliefs among vegans as well. This is an important point because the vegan diet is our point of discussion here, not their philosophies.

Why Vegan Diets are Effective in Weight Loss

While the keto diet focuses mainly on eating fats and proteins, the vegan diet tries to eliminate the same things in their diet. Yet both are effective at weight loss.

A research paper published in 2015 in the Nutrition Journal found that vegans tend to have a lower Body Mass Index (BMI), which is the weight to height ratio of a person. There are also numerous studies that have directly correlating weight loss to a vegan diet.

This is due to the focus on vegetables, fruit, and whole grain which are low in carbohydrates and sugars, and helps the body to burn fat. Controlling sugar and carb intake is the key here, as they cause the release of insulin which limits the body's ability to burn fat.

The OMAD Vegan Diet

The vegan diet has been very popular for weight loss and many studies have shown that it is one of the most effective ways to lose weight.

Science Daily found that the vegan diet was twice as effective for weight loss as one that included meat.

In a recent study published by Science Daily, it was found that vegan diets were much more effective for losing weight than those that included meat.

In fact, the study found that sticking to this type of diet was twice as effective for weight loss, meaning that you would lose double the weight you would if you ate meat while on a diet.

While those who eat animal-based products may find it easier to meet their protein intake needs, there are many other types of foods that you can enjoy while on a vegan diet.

As always, you need to speak with a doctor before deciding to change your diet. If you are introducing the OMAD diet and the vegan diet, you may also want to consider taking this transition in steps to allow your body to acclimatize to the changes.

Aside from the Rule of Four "Ones" which is a standard for all OMAD diets, you should be aware of a few more things when adding veganism as well.

- *Have Variety in Your Meals* - There are many substitutes for non vegan food, and you should experiment with different flavors to enjoy your food more.
- *Choose Umami* - Umami is a category of food taste found in glutamate, a type of amino acid. It is commonly found in meat, but can also be found in mushrooms, onions, and tomatoes.
- *Include Fat* - While animal fat may be off limits to a vegan, avocados, chia seeds, olive oil, and dark chocolate are sources which can be eaten on a vegan diet.
- *Supplement* - There are a number of vitamins and minerals that are not readily available in the vegan diet, so be sure to supplement your food.

Benefits of the Vegan Diet

As we can see from the above section, going vegan will do your body and general health a lot of good. Vegan and vegetarian diets are generally more healthy than other diets, especially if you are looking to lose weight. However, like all diets they have their inherent risks as well.

The study "Nutritional Update for Physicians: Plant-Based Diets" analyzed hundreds of different surveys and found a broad and engaging array of health benefits of a vegan diet.

There are many studies on vegan diets that have found they are high in vitamins C and E, iron, folic acid, fiber, and magnesium, and are naturally healthier than meat-focused diets. The positive results can be summed up as:

Manage weight gain – Vegan diets were found to manage weight gain, as well as speed up weight loss. That's because it naturally balances blood sugar and eliminates problematic fats from your diet.

Manage blood sugar – A vegan diet help to minimize blood guar levels and reduce the insulin in your body. A vegan diet was shown to reduce A1C (average blood sugar levels over 3 months) levels by more than three times the reduction when following the guidelines of the American Diabetes Association (ADA).

Reduced risk of heart disease – Vegas are found to have a 73 percent lower risk of coronary problems. However, this is only true if you avoid refined grains, and processed sugars as well as saturated fat (which vegans already cut out from their diet). Eating nuts also helps to reduce the risk of heart diseases.

Risks of the Vegan Diet

The risks of eating a vegan diet may sound serious, much more serious than a meat based diet. A study, titled "Adherence to Nutrition Recommendations, Use of Supplements Essential for Vegans," found that vegans are generally lacking certain minerals and vitamins in their diet. The consequences of which are an eventual breakdown of the body's functions.

The good news is that most of these risks can be mitigated by taking dietary supplements.

Slow muscle development – Vegans may experience slow muscle development, or long recovery times after working out at the gym. Younger vegans may also experience a slower growth. This is largely due to low levels of protein in their diet.

Weak nervous system – This may appear as anemia, numbness in fingers and toes, fatigue, or dizziness. Prolonged, it may result in permanent damage to the nervous system, and it is largely due to a lack of vitamin B12 which is commonly found in fish and red meat. Older vegans are more susceptible to this.

Hair loss and brittle nails – Dull, lifeless hair that falls off easily and brittle nails that peel off or chip easily are signs of a lack in Omega 3 acids. This is commonly found in fatty fish. Although you can supplement with plat based alternatives like flax seeds and walnuts, they are agreed to be less effective than fish oils.

Weakness and fatigue – Extreme fatigue, weakness, pale skin, headaches, brittle nails, and hair loss may also point to a deficiency in iron. As with Omega 3 acids, they are found in animal protein, and although there are plant based options they are generally not as effective.

Skin problems – Dry skin, eczema, oral ulcers, and hair loss are signs of a Zinc deficiency. They may escalate to more serious issues such as psychological disorders, pregnancy complication in women, and a weak immune system (which will lead to infections which can be fatal).

Brittle bones and joints – The lack of dairy in your diet will make fractures and joint injuries more likely. Calcium deficiency can lead to osteoporosis as you age.

What Supplements are Needed for a Vegan OMAD Diet?

As seen in the previous section, the risks of lacking certain vitamins and minerals are quite severe and vegans need to supplement their daily meals. The recommended daily supplements for a vegan to take are:

Vitamin B12 - This is an essential vitamin because it improves the strength of your body's nervous system and helps make your blood cells healthier. Unfortunately, vegans often suffer from a deficiency of this vitamin.

Vitamin D - This is essential not only for its many benefits but also for the way it helps you absorb other types of vitamins. Its primary purpose is to help your stomach digest and absorb calcium and phosphorous.

Long-Chain Omega-3S - This supplement may provide you with many benefits for your heart. They are also considered to be essential for various other health processes and may improve your overall mental health. While these findings are not conclusive and need more verification, a number of experts in the medical community believe they are accurate.

Iodine - This is meant to keep your thyroid healthy, which controls your metabolism. While experts believe that iodine is deficient in many people around the world, vegans have been found to have half the blood iodine levels of non vegans.

Iron - This is a mineral that is necessary for producing healthy DNA and red blood cells. It is also used to carry oxygen in your blood, and improves metabolism. There is Heme iron which is from meats and chese, and non-heme iron which comes from fruit and vegetables.

Calcium - This is the most important vitamin for your bone health. A lack of calcium can result in weak bones, and in the long term could result in osteoporosis.

Zinc - This is meant to improve your stool density, boost memory, increase healing, manage aging, and improve fertility. However, it is an issue for vegans because foods that contain zinc are primarily based in animal products.

Chapter 10: OMAD Success Stories

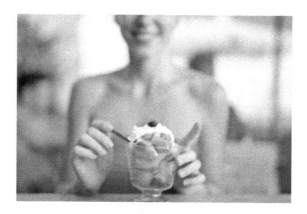

Making a change to your lifestyle is never easy, and we all have our own reasons that we succeed or fail. However, sometimes all we need is someone who has achieved our goals to show us it is possible. Just like the four minute mile.

The four minute mile was a barrier that seemed impossible and it stood for decades. No matter how hard athletes tried to challenge it, the four minute mile remained unbroken. It was a daunting limitation that was as much psychological as it was physical. When Roger Bannister broke that barrier in 1954, many athletes followed closely behind. Today, over 1,400 athletes have conquered that barrier which was once thought of as impossible.

Similarly, I am sharing these stories that come from a diverse group of people, who like you have tried to lose weight but with one difference.. they have already succeeded with the OMAD diet. Their names and identities have been changed, but I hope their stories inspire you all the same to break through your barriers.

"From my own experience, eating more meals leads to me putting on weight and having less of an appetite. I ate because it was meal times. When I started eating only when I was really hungry and I am now eating two meals a day. I have lost body fat, about 18 pounds in the last few weeks. I also feel much better now." Elle D.

 "I'm really excited about this. I've lost 10 pounds in 20 days. It hasn't been that hard to go to one meal as I drink lots of water and my work keeps me really busy. I hardly feel hungry at all." Sienna W.

"I starting eating OMAD a year ago and I have lost 50 pounds and I am now at a healthy weight. At the beginning I was skeptical, but it works. It took a lot of willpower for me as I enjoy snacking, but after a month I got used to it. I was slightly overweight, but I can say this diet has changed my life." Alvaro P

"I started at 350 pounds and I only had one meal a day. No snacks, but I ate whatever I wanted. As I lost weight, I found that I crave junk food less and less, and now I have lost almost 150 pounds. This plan works!" Todd D.

"I am a diabetic, and lost 22 pounds in just over a month simply by following this diet. My blood glucose is better controlled now even though I eat a really big dinner, which is my only meal. The only thing I try to avoid is processed sugars." Cindy V.

"I've tried many diets, but the only one that has helped me lose weight successfully is by eating one meal a day. When I switched to one meal a day I feel I have more energy, and I'm less hungry and I sleep better. The first month I lose 15 pounds, and now I have lost a total of 56 pounds." Rebecca B.

"This is the best diet I've ever done. I have lost a total of 83 pounds on OMAD. When I going to the gym and exercising every day, I only lost 1 pound a week at most. I feel much healthier and more fit now. I only eat one meal twice a week when I'm not exercising, and I'm at the gym the other 5 days." Samson P.

"On one meal a day I'm less hungry than I was when I used to eat and snack throughout the day. Generally, I am able to stick to the diet, but I take a [Energy Drink Brand] if I need a boost during the day." Dan F.

"When I was doing intermittent fasting I was always hungry and thinking about food all day long and had trouble controlling my meals. I would eat a large meal in the afternoon, and be too full for dinner, and my eating window would close. This gave me a lot of trouble sleeping. Now I am a week on one meal a day and I find it surprisingly easy, and I am also on keto. I am still very hungry in the morning, but drinking coffee makes me feel much better." Jacob R.

"I tried eating six meals every two to three hours on my doctor's advice, but it was so hard to stay on schedule. I missed so many meals because of work, and I was never full. I read about the benefits of fasting and with another doctor's help I moved to OMAD. I feel hungry less often now and feel a lot better! Do what works for you, despite the fads." Anna B.

"I lost almost 100 pounds in one year! As the fat guy all my life it is hard to believe that there would come a day when I would be normal. I feel like I am a new person, but I still get to eat all my favorite food. It's like the best of both worlds." Kevin S.

"I eat my meal in a very short window of 30 minutes, and I eat my standard meal which can be anything I want. As a bonus, I finish with something sweet, like an ice cream or a soda. Still I have managed to lose about 10 pounds a month over the last 3 months and look great." Kimberly B.

"I have been eating one meal a day for a year and have lost over 70 pounds. I have tried many diets, but the is the only method that I can follow long term. It's not much of a diet, it's more of a lifestyle. Once I got used to it, eating OMAD is easy." Tony J.

"I have been trying to lose weight for many years by eating just enough to satisfy my appetite whenever I was hungry. I always made healthy food choices, but I was always hungry. This made me anxious, light-headed, and cranky all the time. I also got lethargic in the afternoons and had trouble concentrating. But after I cut out snacks and ate one meal a day, my blood sugar has improved. I am currently eating two meals a day, and have lost 15 pounds." Leslie A.

"I have struggled with dieting for years. I have tried everything. I couldn't stick to any diet and I felt like I would be fat forever. Then I started eating one meal a day. I dropped 12 pounds in my first month alone and I am amazed. The best part is that after the first week I never felt hungry, and I had the freedom to eat what I liked." Christian D.

"I have been eating one meal a day for 6 months and lost 74 pounds. I'm still motivated to keep up this diet because I don't have to plan my meals, count calories, or change my diet. My blood sugar doesn't spike, and I can eat what I want, and I drink lots of water during the day." Vincent M.

"After trying so many diets I was going to give up, but this actually works! I have lost over 25 pounds in three months, and I am at my ideal weight now on OMAD." Sarah W.

BUTTERFINGER PIE

Serves: 8-12

Prep Time: 15 Minutes

Cook Time: 35 Minutes

Total Time: 50 Minutes

INGREDIENTS

pastry sheets

1 package cream cheese

1 tsp vanilla extract

¼ cup peanut butter

1 cup powdered sugar (to decorate)

2 cups Butterfinger candy bars

8 oz whipped topping

DIRECTIONS

1.Line a pie plate or pie form with pastry and cover the edges of the plate depending on your preference

2.In a bowl combine all pie ingredients together and mix well

3.Pour the mixture over the pastry

4.Bake at 400-425 F for 25-30 minutes or until golden brown

5.When ready remove from the oven and let it rest for 15 minutes

STRAWBERRY PIE

Serves: 8-12

Prep Time: 15 Minutes

Cook Time: 35 Minutes

Total Time: 50 Minutes

INGREDIENTS

pastry sheets

1,5 lb. strawberries

1 cup powdered sugar

2 tablespoons cornstarch

1 tablespoon lime juice

1 tsp vanilla extract

2 eggs

2 tablespoons butter

DIRECTIONS

1. Line a pie plate or pie form with pastry and cover the edges of the plate depending on your preference

2.In a bowl combine all pie ingredients together and mix well

3.Pour the mixture over the pastry

4.Bake at 400-425 F for 25-30 minutes or until golden brown

5.When ready remove from the oven and let it rest for 15 minutes

BLUEBERRY PIE

Serves: 8-12

Prep Time: 15 Minutes

Cook Time: 35 Minutes

Total Time: 50 Minutes

INGREDIENTS

pastry sheets

¼ tsp lavender

1 cup brown sugar

4-5 cups blueberries

1 tablespoon lemon juice

1 cup almonds

2 tablespoons butter

DIRECTIONS

1.Line a pie plate or pie form with pastry and cover the edges of the plate depending on your preference

2.In a bowl combine all pie ingredients together and mix well

3.Pour the mixture over the pastry

4.Bake at 400-425 F for 25-30 minutes or until golden brown

5.When ready remove from the oven and let it rest for 15 minutes

GINGER-OAT SMOOTHIE

Serves: 1

Prep Time: 5 Minutes

Cook Time: 5 Minutes

Total Time: 10 Minutes

INGREDIENTS

½ cup oats

¼ cup blueberries

¼ cup vanilla yogurt

1 cup ice

¼ tsp ginger

DIRECTIONS

1.   In a blender place all ingredients and blend until smooth

2.   Pour smoothie in a glass and serve

PUMPKIN SMOOTHIE

Serves: 1

Prep Time: 5 Minutes

Cook Time: 5 Minutes

Total Time: 10 Minutes

INGREDIENTS

1 cup ice

1 cup almond milk

½ cup pumpkin puree

1 tsp honey

DIRECTIONS

1.In a blender place all ingredients and blend until smooth

2.Pour smoothie in a glass and serve

GREEN SMOOTHIE

Serves: 1

Prep Time: 5 Minutes

Cook Time: 5 Minutes

Total Time: 10 Minutes

INGREDIENTS

1 cup kale

1 celery

1 banana

1 cup apple juice

1 cup ice

DIRECTIONS

1.In a blender place all ingredients and blend until smooth

2.Pour smoothie in a glass and serve

MANGO SMOOTHIE

Serves: 1

Prep Time: 5 Minutes

Cook Time: 5 Minutes

Total Time: 10 Minutes

INGREDIENTS

1 cup mango

½ cup coconut milk

1 cup ice

½ cup vanilla yogurt

1 tsp honey

DIRECTIONS

1.In a blender place all ingredients and blend until smooth

2.Pour smoothie in a glass and serve

PINEAPPLE SMOOTHIE

Serves: 1

Prep Time: 5 Minutes

Cook Time: 5 Minutes

Total Time: 10 Minutes

INGREDIENTS

1 cup pineapple

1 cup ice

1 orange juice

½ cup carrot

1 banana

DIRECTIONS

1.In a blender place all ingredients and blend until smooth

2.Pour smoothie in a glass and serve

CASHEW SMOOTHIE

Serves: 1

Prep Time: 5 Minutes

Cook Time: 5 Minutes

Total Time: 10 Minutes

INGREDIENTS

1 cup cashews

1 cup ice

1 banana

1 tablespoon honey

DIRECTIONS

1.In a blender place all ingredients and blend until smooth

2.Pour smoothie in a glass and serve

NUT SMOOTHIE

Serves: 1

Prep Time: 5 Minutes

Cook Time: 5 Minutes

Total Time: 10 Minutes

INGREDIENTS

1 cup coconut milk

1 cup raspberries

1 banana

1 tablespoon peanut butter

1 tsp agave nectar

DIRECTIONS

1.In a blender place all ingredients and blend until smooth

2.Pour smoothie in a glass and serve

STRAWBERRY SMOOTHIE

Serves: 1

Prep Time: 5 Minutes

Cook Time: 5 Minutes

Total Time: 10 Minutes

INGREDIENTS

1 cup strawberries

1 cup Greek Yoghurt

½ cup orange juice

1 tsp honey

1 tablespoon flaxseed meal

DIRECTIONS

1.In a blender place all ingredients and blend until smooth

2.Pour smoothie in a glass and serve

SPINACH & GRAPE SMOOTHIE

Serves: 1

Prep Time: 5 Minutes

Cook Time: 5 Minutes

Total Time: 10 Minutes

INGREDIENTS

1 cup grapes

1 cup baby spinach

1 cup ice

1 cup almond milk

DIRECTIONS

1.In a blender place all ingredients and blend until smooth

2.Pour smoothie in a glass and serve

ICE-CREAM RECIPES

SAFFRON ICE-CREAM

Serves: 6-8

Prep Time: 15 Minutes

Cook Time: 15 Minutes

Total Time: 30 Minutes

INGREDIENTS

4 egg yolks

1 cup heavy cream

1 cup milk

½ cup brown sugar

1 tsp saffron

1 tsp vanilla extract

DIRECTIONS

1.In a saucepan whisk together all ingredients

2.Mix until bubbly

3.Strain into a bowl and cool

4.Whisk in favorite fruits and mix well

5.Cover and refrigerate for 2-3 hours

6.Pour mixture in the ice-cream maker and follow manufacturer instructions

7.Serve when ready

PISTACHIOS ICE-CREAM

Serves: 6-8

Prep Time: 15 Minutes

Cook Time: 15 Minutes

Total Time: 30 Minutes

INGREDIENTS

4 egg yolks

1 cup heavy cream

1 cup milk

1 cup sugar

1 vanilla bean

1 tsp almond extract

1 cup cherries

½ cup pistachios

DIRECTIONS

1.In a saucepan whisk together all ingredients

2.Mix until bubbly

3.Strain into a bowl and cool

4.Whisk in favorite fruits and mix well

5.Cover and refrigerate for 2-3 hours

6.Pour mixture in the ice-cream maker and follow manufacturer instructions

VANILLA ICE-CREAM

Serves: 6-8

Prep Time: 15 Minutes

Cook Time: 15 Minutes

Total Time: 30 Minutes

INGREDIENTS

1 cup milk

1 tablespoon cornstarch

1 oz. cream cheese

1 cup heavy cream

1 cup brown sugar

1 tablespoon corn syrup

1 vanilla bean

DIRECTIONS

1.In a saucepan whisk together all ingredients

2.Mix until bubbly

3.Strain into a bowl and cool

4.Whisk in favorite fruits and mix well

5.Cover and refrigerate for 2-3 hours

6.Pour mixture in the ice-cream maker and follow manufacturer instructions

7.Serve when ready

SPICY SHRIMP STIR FRY

Serves: 1

Prep Time: 10 Minutes

Cook Time: 10 Minutes

Total Time: 20 Minutes

INGREDIENTS

1 orange

Cayenne powder

3 oz shrimp

Ginger powder

4 tbs vegetable stock

Curry powder

25 cups red onion

1 cup cabbage

Garlic powder

DIRECTIONS

1.Coat the shrimp in the seasonings.

2.Pour the broth into a pan, then add cabbage, onion, and shrimp.

3.Cook until the shrimp turns pink.

4.Serve topped with orange juice and orange slices.

ARTICHOKE AND SPINACH PIZZA

Serves: 6-8

Prep Time: 10 Minutes

Cook Time: 15 Minutes

Total Time: 25 Minutes

INGREDIENTS

1 pizza crust

1 garlic clove

½ lb. spinach

½ lb. soft cheese

2 oz. artichoke hearts

1 cup mozzarella cheese

1 tablespoon olive oil

DIRECTIONS

1.Spread tomato sauce on the pizza crust

2.Place all the toppings on the pizza crust

3.Bake the pizza at 425 F for 12-15 minutes

4.When ready remove pizza from the oven and serve

MINT PIZZA

Serves: 6-8

Prep Time: 10 Minutes

Cook Time: 15 Minutes

Total Time: 25 Minutes

INGREDIENTS

1 pizza crust

1 olive oil

1 garlic clove

1 cup mozzarella cheese

2 oz. mint

2 courgettes

DIRECTIONS

1.Spread tomato sauce on the pizza crust

2.Place all the toppings on the pizza crust

3.Bake the pizza at 425 F for 12-15 minutes

4.When ready remove pizza from the oven and serve

SAUSAGE PIZZA

Serves: 6-8

Prep Time: 10 Minutes

Cook Time: 15 Minutes

Total Time: 25 Minutes

INGREDIENTS

2 pork sausages

1 tablespoon olive oil

2 garlic cloves

1 tsp fennel seeds

½ lb. ricotta

1 cup mozzarella cheese

1 oz. parmesan cheese

1 pizza crust

DIRECTIONS

1.Spread tomato sauce on the pizza crust

2.Place all the toppings on the pizza crust

3.Bake the pizza at 425 F for 12-15 minutes

4.When ready remove pizza from the oven and serve

BEEF & BROCCOLI STIR FRY

Serves: 4

Prep Time: 10 Minutes

Cook Time: 30 Minutes

Total Time: 40 Minutes

INGREDIENTS

2 cloves garlic

½ lb Beef Sirloin steaks

Chicken broth

2 tbs liquid Aminos

1 tsp onion powder

1 tbs parsley

2 cups broccoli florets

DIRECTIONS

1.Sauté the beef in a few tbs of chicken broth until brown.

2.Add onion powder, garlic, broccoli, liquid aminos and parsley.

3.Saute until well done.

4.Serve immediately.

GINGER CHICKEN SOUP

Serves: 1

Prep Time: 5 Minutes

Cook Time: 15 Minutes

Total Time: 20 Minutes

INGREDIENTS

2 cloves garlic

Salt

Pepper

3 stalks celery

3 oz chicken tenders

4 cups chicken broth

4 slices ginger

DIRECTIONS

1.Bring the broth to a boil.

2.Add the garlic, ginger, and celery.

3.Simmer for 5 minutes.

4.Add in the chicken and boil for 10 more minutes.

5.Season with salt and pepper.

6.Serve immediately.

CILANTRO SKEWERS

Serves: 1

Prep Time: 20 Minutes

Cook Time: 120 Minutes

Total Time: 140 Minutes

INGREDIENTS

Cherry tomatoes

Red pepper flakes

Salt

Pepper

2 tbs lemon juice

Cilantro

100g shrimp

DIRECTIONS

1.Mix the cilantro, red pepper flakes, salt, pepper and shrimp together.

2.Marinade for at least 2 hours.

3.Place on skewers alternating with tomatoes.

4.Cook on a barbeque.

5.Season with salt and pepper.

6.Serve immediately.

CURRY SHRIMP

Serves: 14

Prep Time: 10 Minutes

Cook Time: 10 Minutes

Total Time: 20 Minutes

INGREDIENTS

1/8 cup water

100g shrimp

1 onion

Pepper

1/ tsp curry powder

¼ tsp cumin

Salt

4 garlic cloves

DIRECTIONS

1.Cook the garlic and onion until translucent.

2.Add in the shrimp, seasonings and water.

3.Cook until done.

4.Serve immediately.

ORANGE ROUGHY

Serves: 1

Prep Time: 10 Minutes

Cook Time: 15 Minutes

Total Time: 25 Minutes

INGREDIENTS

100g orange roughy fillet

2 tbs lemon juice

1 tsp thyme

1 tsp rosemary

¼ tsp onion powder

Salt

Pepper

DIRECTIONS

1.Place the ingredients in a baking dish and cover with tin foil.

2.Bake at 350F for 15 minutes.

3.Serve hot.

LEMON TILAPIA

Serves: 1

Prep Time: 10 Minutes

Cook Time: 20 Minutes

Total Time: 30 Minutes

INGREDIENTS

¼ cup lemon juice

1 lemon zest

100g tilapia

1 tbs onion

1 tsp dill

Salt

Pepper

DIRECTIONS

1.Place the ingredients in a tin foil, then wrap them up.

2.Cook on a grill until done

3.Serve when ready

MEDITERRANEAN SEA BASS

Serves: 1

Prep Time: 10 Minutes

Cook Time: 10 Minutes

Total Time: 20 Minutes

INGREDIENTS

100g sea Bass

2 cloves garlic

1 lemon juice

1 lemon zest

1 tbs onion

½ tsp parsley

Salt

Pepper

DIRECTIONS

1.Place the ingredients in a tin foil bag.

2.Cook on the barbeque for 10 minutes.

3.Serve topped with fresh parsley.

WASABI WHITEFISH

Serves: 1

Prep Time: 10 Minutes

Cook Time: 5 Minutes

Total Time: 15 Minutes

INGREDIENTS

½ tsp ginger

100g whitefish

1 tbs mustard

1 tsp wasabi powder

DIRECTIONS

1.Mix the mustard with the wasabi powder.

2.Add the ginger.

3.Coat the fish with the mixture.

4.Allow to sit for at least half an hour.

5.Grill for 5 minutes.

6.Serve hot.

CAJUN CHICKEN

Serves: 1

Prep Time: 5 Minutes

Cook Time: 25 Minutes

Total Time: 30 Minutes

INGREDIENTS

½ tbs milk

½ tsp Cajun seasoning

100g chicken

DIRECTIONS

1.Preheat the oven to 350F.

2.Coat the chicken with milk.

3.Sprinkle with Cajun seasoning.

4.Bake for 25 minutes.

5.Serve immediately.

BASIL CHICKEN SANDWICH

Serves: 1

Prep Time: 5 Minutes

Cook Time: 0 Minutes

Total Time: 5 Minutes

INGREDIENTS

½ tomato

1 toast

100g chicken

Basil

Salt

Pepper

DIRECTIONS

1.Cook the chicken, allow to chill, then shred.

2.Arrange the ingredients on top of the toast.

3.Serve immediately.

MARINARA CHICKEN

Serves: 1

Prep Time: 10 Minutes

Cook Time: 25 Minutes

Total Time: 35 Minutes

INGREDIENTS

½ tsp oregano

Parsley

100g chicken

1 toast

½ tsp basil

3 garlic cloves

2 tsp onion

Salt

Pepper

DIRECTIONS

1.Crush the toast and combine with oregano, basil, salt, and pepper.

2.Coat the chicken with the mixture and place in a casserole dish.

3.Cook covered for 25 minutes at 375F.

4.Serve topped with marinara sauce and parsley.

EDAMAME FRITATTA

Serves: 2

Prep Time: 10 Minutes

Cook Time: 20 Minutes

Total Time: 30 Minutes

INGREDIENTS

1 cup edamame

1 tablespoon olive oil

½ red onion

2 eggs

¼ tsp salt

2 oz. cheddar cheese

1 garlic clove

¼ tsp dill

DIRECTIONS

1.In a bowl whisk eggs with salt and cheese

2.In a frying pan heat olive oil and pour egg mixture

3.Add remaining ingredients and mix well

4.Serve when ready

LEEKS FRITATTA

Serves: 2

Prep Time: 10 Minutes

Cook Time: 20 Minutes

Total Time: 30 Minutes

INGREDIENTS

½ lb. leek

1 tablespoon olive oil

½ red onion

¼ tsp salt

2 eggs

2 oz. cheddar cheese

1 garlic clove

¼ tsp dill

DIRECTIONS

1.In a bowl whisk eggs with salt and cheese

2.In a frying pan heat olive oil and pour egg mixture

3.Add remaining ingredients and mix well

4.Serve when ready

MUSHROOM FRITATTA

Serves: 2

Prep Time: 10 Minutes

Cook Time: 20 Minutes

Total Time: 30 Minutes

INGREDIENTS

½ lb. mushrooms

1 tablespoon olive oil

½ red onion

¼ tsp salt

2 eggs

2 oz. cheddar cheese

1 garlic clove

¼ tsp dill

DIRECTIONS

1.In a bowl whisk eggs with salt and cheese

2.In a frying pan heat olive oil and pour egg mixture

3.Add remaining ingredients and mix well

4.Serve when ready

Conclusion

Congratulations for making it to the end and thank you for taking the time to read this book!

Hopefully you now have a good idea of what the OMAD diet is and whether it is for you, even if you work out, or have dietary restrictions like keto or veganism, OMAD can work for you. Otherwise you may prefer to choose a less demanding regime, but incorporate fasting into your daily routines as a "baby step".

The next step then is to consult with your doctor, begin your meal planning, and slowly prepare to cut your meals down to one. The OMAD diet does not have to be a struggle if you understand what to expect and make your preparations accordingly.

Whether you are looking to lose weight, gain muscle, or have a healthier lifestyle, if you approach OMAD with a solid plan and have the motivation and determination to follow through, you can live a healthy fulfilling life with one meal a day. Lots of people have already done it.

CPSIA information can be obtained
at www.ICGtesting.com
Printed in the USA
BVHW051727010323
659501BV00023B/455